Chasing
The Elusive
Work-Life Balance

FOR THE WORKING SINGAPOREAN

Chasing
The Elusive
Work-Life Balance

FOR THE WORKING SINGAPOREAN

Written by
Muhamad Hamim Bin Abdul Rahim

Edited by
Nuraisha Teng

Illustration by
Maryam Binte Muhamad Hamim

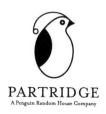

PARTRIDGE
A Penguin Random House Company

To order additional copies of this book, contact
Toll Free 800 101 2657 (Singapore)
Toll Free 1 800 81 7340 (Malaysia)
orders.singapore@partridgepublishing.com

www.facebook.com/chasingtheelusive
www.partridgepublishing.com/singapore

Contents

To my children,
Maryam, Hakiim, Matiin, Lathiif and Marhamah,

I want to be the best father I can be. I hope this book will inspire you to do the things your would have never thought possible and always remember that you are all special in your own ways with special gifts that you have developed with hard work. Lastly, always believe that you are destined to do good, overcome evil and improve the lives of the less fortunate.

To my wife
Fatimah Sawifi,

You are my rock, my listening post, my sponge, my blind spot mirror and a plaster for my wound. You are the first I look for to share my joy and my disappointments in life. Without you, I am a sail without the wind, a flag without a post and a spring without a force. I love you sayang.

To my friends and readers

To all those seeking to strike a balance between career and personal life, my friends, my colleagues and my course mates, thank you for spurring me on with your encouraging words.

Introduction

Work life balance has been getting quite a fair share of attention lately here in Singapore, so much so that it has become a tag phrase. At the various Singapore Conversations, participants regularly bring up topics related to improving the quality of life given that the life here is fast paced and stressful. The term work-life balance can almost be used synonymously with slowing down, relaxing, stopping and smelling the roses etc. This is rightfully so because many of us have experienced some sort of burnout at work. Yet, on the other side of the spectrum, experts have observed that some of us have interpreted this term in a way that we have taken a more precautionary approach to career and life, so much so that we have made a decision not to work hard and open the door of opportunity when it comes knocking just so we can breathe better in our personal space. Prime Minister Lee Hsien Loong, in a televised forum in September 2013, warned Singaporeans that such attitude can result in our competitors 'stealing lunches' from our own plates.

So, is work life balance a myth as some writers on this topic have called it? Is it achievable and realistic? Can we continue to give our best or commit to doing our best in our career and yet have a fulfilling personal life? This is what this book aims to answer. It will show how we can adopt simple healthy practices with the right attitude and motivation which will enable us to enhance and boost our personal lives yet, continue to give quality performance at work. To add greater dimension to the issue of work life balance, a family perspective will be included too. So I hope this book will convince you that work life balance can be achieved even in a fast-paced society like ours and enable all of us to improve the quality of our lives. Since my expertise is in the area of physical well-being, this book will have greater detail on physical health and fitness for example weight management and fitness improvement. In these pages, you will also be able to find how to adopt the right motivation to fuel the changes you may want to make.

About the Author

Muhamad Hamim is a Senior Physical Education teacher with the Ministry of Education, Singapore. He graduated from the School of Physical Education and Sports Science from the National Institute of Education, Nanyang Technological University in 1993 with a diploma and taught in a primary school for six years. He then furthered his studies at Loughborough University in the United Kingdom where he graduated with second upper class honours. Following that, he taught at a secondary school and a junior college. He has been a teacher for 21 years. Health Education is his passion and Physical Education for life is his personal motto. He has been on work attachments to the Health Promotion Board and Alexandra Hospital (Weight Management Centre) and conducted talks, workshops and presentations at school, cluster and national levels. He is married and has five school going children. He is an avid triathlete and finds time to train regularly despite his busy career and family life. This was not the case previously where he led a largely sedentary lifestyle and didn't observe a healthy diet. His turning point came when he was in his mid-thirties. He was told that he had high cholesterol and had to take medication for the rest of his life. From that point onwards he managed to turn around and changed his lifestyle to a healthier one. It had a profound effect on not only him but the people around him. He made it a personal mission to share this joy with as many people as he knows and he hopes that by penning his method and sharing it, more people can experience the positive impact of a healthier lifestyle. He believes that balancing work and family life is possible and important.

Foreword

Hamim has tackled a common-yet-challenging aspect of our lives, achieving a healthy work-life balance. But he has made use of old and new science to make this an enjoyable read. It is made even more interesting because local as well as world data has been used to argue the case for a better work-life balance.

Best of all there is so much practical advice simply because Hamim started living his present lifestyle at the critical mid-30s and has shown that it can be done. In his book, he gives practical advice of making simple modifications to our lifestyle and explains how each strategy helps. He also teaches how to develop the right attitude and motivation which will enable us to enhance and boost our personal lives and most importantly continue to give quality performance at work.

Teens in schools, tertiary students who are forever pressured for time, young and older working adults and retirees should read this simply and yet accurately written book.

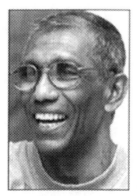

Mr C Kunalan
Olympian, coach, teacher, lecturer, mentor,
a dedicated father & a loving husband

"Always trying to maintain some fitness level. Not easy but we have to make it part of our daily routine. No matter what. Fitness first or Family first? Or Finance first? Tough!!"

Chapter 1

The DRESS UP Approach
to Work-life Balance

Let's begin, with the end in mind, literally, by answering a simple question. If we can choose the way we die, how would it be? Fifteen years ago, one of my university lecturers said that if he could choose a method to die, he would like his death to be a sudden one. He illustrated this by drawing an imaginary graph in the air with his hands. He straightened his fingers, palm facing downwards and moved it from left to right in front of his chest. At the end of it, he turned his palm inward and brought his hands down as if he was slicing a cake. He explained that one would be healthy throughout his life before suddenly dying. He drew another imaginary graph. This time, it goes diagonally down. The second graph means one would be experiencing deteriorating health as he or she ages prior to death, he asserted. Can his assertion be substantiated? Indeed so. A Straits Times report in 2007 cited that Singaporeans live longer but suffer eight years of poor health. Globally, Dailymail.co.uk reports that from 1990 to 2010, life expectancy has risen from 59 to 70 years old but it is accompanied by an increase in the number of years people live with chronic diseases such as back pain, diabetes, arthritis and depression. I am sure all of us want to live longer with good health, unburdened by the plausible need to keep seeing a doctor or relying on medication or undergo medical treatment in hopes to cure ourselves. The scenario paints a gloomy picture where we can no longer cope with living with chronic or debilitating medical condition, resulting in relying on loved ones to care for us.

But just how important is work-life balance to the Singaporean worker? Well, a survey commissioned by The Straits Times recorded the responses of 501 Singapore residents on what they value most about their job. Each respondent was tasked to rank these six items in order of importance;

- good pay,
- good work-life balance,
- good bosses/colleagues,
- opportunities for career advancement,
- personally fulfilling and
- meaningful and convenience (near home, easy to travel to).

The findings, published in the The Straits Times on 3 August 2013 showed that across the ages of 16 to 62, work-life balance was placed second. Those in the ages of 30 to 40 ranked it first. Work-life balance seems to fall behind good pay but only slightly, where the latter positioned itself as the top choice for those in the 20s, 40s and 50s. What this means is that workers value work-life balance almost as much as the pay. In one group, the 30s, work-life balance was even more important. They were willing to be paid less to have greater work-life balance. The reasons were not clearly discussed but it is definitely obvious among my peers. Into their mid-thirties, with children to tend to, some female officers opted to leave the service or take a pay cut for flexible working arrangements just to spend more time raising their children. This meant living with just one breadwinner in the family hence a lower family income.

The Definition and Components of Health

Work-life balance has a very strong relationship with health. Thus to understand better, we need to explore the issues related to health. The World Health Organization (WHO) defines health as a state of complete physical, mental and social well-being and not merely the absence of disease or infirmity. In order to achieve overall health, or holistic health, one would have to possess the three components of health which is physical, mental and social. The development of these three components, in many occasions, may overlap and complement each other. This is good news for sure. For example a group of friends engaging in a game of bowling would encompass all three aspects of health. The physical act of bowling the ball towards the pins contributes to muscular and bone development. It also develops coordination and balance. Communicating with each other throughout the session develops social health and sharpens social skills. Mental health gets a boost if the player is new to the sports. This is because learning a new skill stimulates the mind and arrests any form of mental degradation. If the game requires team effort in strategizing and calculating scores, the benefits to social and mental health will automatically be further increased. That explains why experts advise exercising in groups because it is more beneficial and the dependency on one another will also mean greater continuity.

The DRESS UP Approach

Over at Boon Lay Secondary School (BLSS) where I teach Physical Education (PE) and promote health to my staff and the community, we have re-packaged the three components of health into something we hope would be more digestible. The term DRESS UP was coined to point out the importance of looking good. But it is not the clothes that should be emphasized. Rather, it is the inside of the person that matters the most because when a person is healthy, the physical appearance would automatically look good and smart. The confidence that comes with a healthy and strong body would also boost a person's confidence and self-esteem. With an overall luminous disposition or aura, one is seen to be attractive. Thus, what is worn on the outside is not as important as what is on the inside, a phrase teachers regularly emphasize to our students.

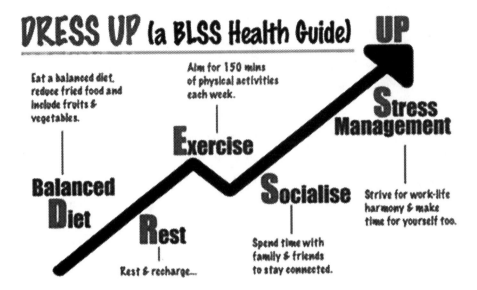

DRESS UP (a BLSS Health Guide) UP

Eat a balanced diet, reduce fried food and include fruits & vegetables.

Aim for 150 mins of physical activities each week.

Exercise

Stress Management

Balanced Diet

Rest

Socialise

Strive for work-life harmony & make time for yourself too.

Rest & recharge...

Spend time with family & friends to stay connected.

This Health Guide - **Dress Up** is the 'how' of healthy living. By following the guide, you can achieve an acceptable level of holistic well-being. You will then look and feel great and smart, thus the word **DRESS**. The word **UP** represents the continuous effort to improve all aspects of health over time.

Boon Lay Secondary School

The first three letters of this acronym, D for diet, R for rest and E for exercise falls under the physical domain while the first S for Socialise is to explore social health and the other S is stress management will look into the mental health domain. In our guide, we recommend eating a balanced diet, reducing the consumption of fried food and to include fruits and vegetable in our daily meals. Rest is important too because it means that we can recover and recharge from the daily stresses of life. For exercise, we recommend clocking 150 hours' worth of physical activity a week. We also included socializing as spending time with family and friends to stay connected. To manage stress while maintaining good mental health, we recommend striving for work-life harmony and making some time for oneself each day. Finally, UP means uniformed progression to indicate that we must always continually improve each of these components so that we do not stagnate as our body tends to adapt to changes all too quickly.

The diagram can be seen on the left. More details of these strategies will be discussed in the ensuing chapters. But before we can flip the pages and learn about what needs to be done to achieve better health, there is actually another factor as important, if not more, that must be set right to ensure greater success. This factor is called motivation.

Motivation

Motivation is what drives us to do something and continue doing it over a period of time. This to me is the most important factor when adopting or developing a new habit. There are many types of motivation but two of the most common is internal and external motivation. While internal motivation is the inner voice in us that tells us what to do like, "I think I will go for a brisk walk in the evening because it is good for my health.", the part where "…it is good for my health." is the internal motivation. It is doing something for the sake of the activity itself and comes from the person. External motivation, however, is quite the opposite. It is doing something because of something else for example, "I think I will go for a brisk walk later in the evening because it will make my husband happy." For this case, the husband can be regarded as the external motivator. To better understand internal and external motivation, I would tell my class this story which I picked up from a talk. There was a group of ruffians who terrorized a shopkeeper every day of the week. They would walk into the shop and mess it up. As they walked out of the shop, they would laugh out loud and warn the shopkeeper against calling the authorities. After a while, the shopkeeper had an idea. The next time the group came, he told them that he would pay them a sum of money to wreck his place. Puzzled but pleasantly surprised, the group of boys did their job and was paid at the end of the carnage. This continued for about a week until the shopkeeper explained to them that business was bad and he wasn't able to pay them anymore for their work but they were welcomed to continue messing up his shop. Upon hearing the news, the leader decided that it was no longer rewarding to continue with the enterprise without any monetary reward and left without ever returning again. Knowingly or unknowingly, the shopkeeper actually shifted the motivation of the group from internal to external. When the group started the activity, it was for its own sake, or for fun as they enjoyed it but as soon as they were paid, the reason for doing it changed to monetary incentive and when that incentive was removed, so was the reason for doing the activity which they enjoyed in the first place. There are many lessons to learn from here. Internal motivation is a stronger force and tends to be more permanent or long-lasting. External motivation can be a strong force, in fact, maybe even stronger than internal at certain point in time. However, its effect does not last as long in most instances. This is especially true when the external motivation or motivator is removed or stopped. Internal and external motivation do not operate in silos. In fact, when we pick up a reason to do something, most of the time it is a combination. But it is useful to consciously stress internal motivation. For example, if we decide to start on a new programme of renewal, where for instance we, adopt a healthy activity like brisk walking, we should ask ourselves what the actual reasons are for doing that. If the reason is simply to improve our health, this is known to be an internal motivator. If the reason is to lose weight so as to look better physically for others to see, then this is seen as an external motivator. These two reasons may be used together but it is important to emphasize that internal motivation should be the main driver as it will ensure greater sustainability. I would like to think that the external motivator is a good starter but internal motivation is the one that sustains one's effort in engaging in the exercise. A very good and strong external motivator, for example, is family and friends. Look at the health tagline adopted by my school to promote health among the students, staff and parents. Can you guess if it is internal or external?

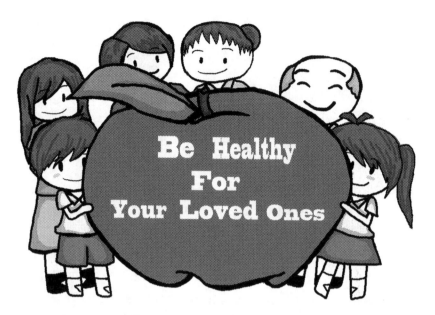

Boon Lay Secondary School

If you chose the latter, then you are right. This tagline was adapted from LTA's EMAS message to motorist to drive safely for our loved ones. It is a strong motivator because many of us would go out of our way for our loved ones to ensure that they are not inconvenienced or even endangered. That however has its own limitations. For all, if not most, in external motivation, when the stimulus is no longer present, then the motivation to continue with the current behavior may stop. For example, Tony has been in a relationship with Lisa for several months now and they both have adopted each other's healthy habits. With Lisa, Tony has introduced salad and fruits into his diet as the former believes in the health benefits of fibre and consumes raw greens and fruits daily. As for Lisa, she started cycling because Tony is an avid cyclist. They would ride on the park connectors in the evenings together regularly. Their love for each other spurred them to leverage on each other's positive health habits and soon they found their body and mind getting stronger and healthier. At this point in time, it would be reasonable to assume that the new dietary habit and the exercise regime Tony and Lisa adopted respectively would continue if the relationship continues. There is therefore the possibility that if the relationship discontinued then the new habits that the couple had adopted may stop. Other examples of external motivation could include

- achieving desired weight (by losing or gaining weight) to look better (for others),
- physical gain such as monetary award, prize, trophy, medals, certificates, etc,
- doing things to please parents or significant others.

As mentioned before, external and internal motivation are useful and important in their own ways. When trying to lose or gain weight, I often offer the advice to focus on improvement in fitness rather than reducing weight. There are several reasons for this. Firstly, losing weight is more often than not, an external motivation because the target weight is achievable or finite and once the target weight is achieved, healthy habits which were previously adopted may not be sustained because we may feel that we are at the end of our journey. Secondly, losing weight may get us fixated on the numbers churned out by the weighing scale each time we step on it. It would be better to focus our attention on how fun, meaningful and beneficial our effort has been so far to be healthier. Thirdly, focusing on fitness gains is better because fitness is infinite and more difficult to achieve and sustain, making it more challenging. What I mean is getting stronger and faster or the physical activity or sports getting easier over time. Take on a fitness test like a 2.4km run or a 2km walk to find out how fit we are and try to sustain over the years. It is not easy and it will require us to sustain our healthy efforts.

Sometimes, I like to sit with my students and ask them why they go to school. I get a myriad of reactions. Some would give me the politically-correct answer that it was for the acquisition of knowledge. Others would say that it was because their parents told them to do so and some because of friends. These are the top three answers I would get. While the first answer falls under internal motivation, the other two are external.

Some people view the three components of health separately. Consider the three types of profiles. One is the lone jogger and dieter. He may possess excellent fitness and medically sound body but lives alone as he is void of friends and ostracized by the family for whatever reasons. His small or non-existent social circle would mean that he would have problems understanding social norms and complying with rules and the law. It may also mean this person may have poor coping skills and time management ability to meet deadlines at work. Second is the friendly colleague or responsible family man or woman who has many social circles. He goes out with different friends or spends dedicated time with family, every day after work and over the weekends ignoring his waistline and deadlines. Sooner or later, the act of ignoring any form of physical activity and diet can cause medical ailments. The daily routines will soon get monotonous and he will notice his work piling up and gets to a point where it creates stress. The third profile is the lone workaholic. He excels at the workplace by taking on many projects and meeting all deadlines. He is hailed as the model worker by his boss or perhaps is the model boss himself, climbing the corporate ladder at any cost. Unfortunately, calls by friends and family to spend time with them fall onto deaf ears and his haphazard diet of take outs and hawker food as well as the absence of any form of physical activity contribute to a growing waistline. As such, his social and physical health worsens as a result of his lifestyle.

Health Screening – The Starting Point

Some people I meet do not like to have their health measured. This is quite understandable as they fear something would be discovered and they cannot continue with their current lifestyle. So for those who have actually taken the step forward to get their health screened, I say to them, "Well done!" And for those who knows they are unhealthy but still underwent the health screening I say to them, "Double well done!" And for those who have not had their health check, may I encourage them to sign up for one as soon as possible or whenever opportunities appear. The wonderful saying of the Chinese Philosopher Lao Tzu captures it all - "The journey of a thousand miles begin with a single step." Knowing our health status must be the first step towards living a healthy lifestyle in many years to come. There is another saying that may be worth surfacing. I remember reading a newspaper article where a father was advising a daughter about her career which goes like, "Don't trouble trouble unless trouble troubles you." It's a wonderful saying which I often use to advise my students who gets themselves in trouble. It is also applicable in the area of health, albeit, in a negative way. This is where one would take action only when ailments are presented before him. For as long as this does not happen, the person remains passive and dormant about his lifestyle. So to me, if trouble is in the form of lifestyle diseases like high blood pressure, it is worth to trouble trouble because if we do not find out, the condition can get worse and when it does rear its ugly head, things can be too late. In this aspect, I prefer the English saying, "prevention is better than cure".

I think we are very lucky in Singapore to have good access to health care. Community centers, the workplace and special health promoting events offer free basic medical screening. The various schemes, financial and manpower support from the Health Promotion Board have made this possible. What are measured at the screening sessions are quite basic. Nonetheless, they are sufficient. These are screening for Body Mass Index or BMI, Blood Pressure, Blood Glucose and Cholesterol levels. Other checks can be conducted at an additional costs. Sometimes organizers will prepare special body scan machines where participants are assessed to know the amount of fats and muscles in their body. More interestingly, these machines are able to verify the person's actual body age, which I personally have come to like. These machine looks like ordinary bathroom scale with flat metal surfaces.

Sending very low electrical current throughout the body, the scale is able to ascertain the amount of muscles and fats found in one's body. From there, it will be able to tell the person's body age. When compared to the actual age of the person, interesting results can be observed. In some cases where the actual body age measured by the machine is found to be higher, the person will profess shock and disbelief after which he or she will make a pledge to make an improvement to his or her health. Those whose body age is younger than their actual age, feels satisfied and vindicated. These body scans are getting more popular and can be found quite easily in major shopping centers, costing around $100. With one of these, one is able to do their own medical health screening which should be done at regular intervals, annually if possible. This would allow the individual to see if intervention measures need to be adopted, for example changing lifestyle to a healthier one or seek medical advice. For those who have been physically dormant for many years, it is advisable to visit a doctor to get medically screened before embarking on an exercise regime. I had mine done before starting on the sports of triathlon after being inactive for more than ten years. Seeing a doctor was not only reassuring for me but for my wife too who was worried I may be exerting beyond what my body can take. Indeed that was money worth spending.

BMI

There are actually many ways or tools to measure one's level of health. The Body Mass Index (BMI) is one which is widely adopted by many health institutions and practitioners due to its ease of measurement. To find out our BMI, we need to know our weight and height. Generally our height doesn't change much between the ages of 20 – 60. What changes the most is our weight. To calculate our BMI, simply measure our weight in kilogram and our height in meters and apply the following formula;

$$weight \div height \times height = BMI$$

For example if my weight is 60kg and my height is 1.65m then my BMI would be

$$60kg \div (1.65m \times 1.65m) = 60kg \div (2.7225m^2)$$
$$= 22kg/m^2$$

$$BMI = 22$$

But what does this all mean; am I healthy? Now we have to look at the value table which is provided by HPB.

ASIAN Values

BMI (kg/m2) for Adults	Health Risk
27.5 and above	High Risk
23 – 27.4	Moderate Risk
18.5 – 22.9	Low Risk (healthy range)
Below 18.5	Risk of nutritional deficiency diseases and osteoporosis

So, my BMI of 22 puts me at the low risk level. However it is at the upper range. One of the interesting observations about BMI is that although I am in the upper range of the low risk category, missing the moderate risk range by just one point, in terms of the way I look, I frequently get comments by friends and relatives saying that I am skinny. This has actually got me to conclude that to be in the healthy range in Singapore and in other Asian communities, one has to appear as such, skinny or lean. But why is this so? To understand this, we need to be aware that these values have actually been revised from the standard values where Caucasians fall into. The standard value can be studied below

International Standard Values

BMI (kg/m2) for Adults	Classification
≥ 30	Obese
≥ 25	Overweight
18.5 – 24.99	Normal Range
< 18.5	Underweight

There are several notable differences in the values table above. Firstly, the descriptors. The international standard table attaches the BMI values to body weight while the Asian values attaches risk level. The latter I feel is better as it implicates diseases, therefore it is more pragmatic. For example, the normal range in the standard table may give the idea that those who are in this category will not be experiencing any form of health related ailments. At about the same standing as the standard value, an Asian would find himself or herself to be at low risk. This is more accurate I think because there are those who actually have good BMI but also have lifestyle diseases such as high blood pressure or high cholesterol levels or both. The second important thing to note about the differences between the two standards is the acceptable level. While the standard one is at 18.5 – 24.9, the Asian equivalent is at 18.5 – 22.9. This discrepancy means that race does dictate whether one is unhealthy or not. For example if a person's BMI is 24 he is considered not healthy if he is an Asian but healthy if he is a Caucasian. Why is there such discrimination? Well, studies showed that Asians have higher proportion of body fat compared to Caucasians of the same age, gender and BMI. They also show that Asians have increased risk for cardiovascular diseases and diabetes even at lower level of BMI. Lately, researchers are also recommending the blacks to use the Asian values due to deteriorating health status. I often wonder why there is such a difference. Why are Caucasians healthier than Asians so much so at the same BMI value, the former has lower risk factor? For this question I had to make my own conclusion which ranges from genetic predisposition to diet. With reference to the latter, I simplified that the Asian diet is higher in fats and cholesterol as compared to Western food. If this argument is not convincing enough, I would like to put forward the idea that Caucasians consumption of vegetables is better. For example, they eat their vegetable raw like in salads. In contrast, Asians tend to cook and even overcook the vegetables. I had the opportunity once to attend a food sampling of potential canteen vendors when I was in the canteen committee in school. There were several candidates and they were given time to prepare their dishes to impress the committee members. One of the candidates I was told was a former chef of a hotel so I was looking forward to tasting his food. It would be great to have a former chef to give quality, value for money food to our students, I thought but I have to remain fair and unbiased too to the rest. But what I saw disturbed me. He cooked a vegetable dish. The vegetable was boiled for some time before it was removed and then cooked again in a broth. Being cooked twice, I wonder how much nutrients and fibre the vegetables can retain. I voiced my concern and my vice –principle who was heading the committee said that was a common cooking method. Luckily the ex-chef was receptive to our concerns and was willing to make adjustments.

BMI Figures and Limitations

The National Health Survey of 2010 reports that 40.1% of Singaporean adults are overweight. This means that for every 5 adults on the street, 2 are overweight. In the UK, the figure is 60.1% while in the USA it is 69.2%. The World Health Organization (WHO) calls obesity, which is the more severe form of overweight, as "one of today's most blatantly visible – yet most neglected – public health problems." It was then labelled a "global epidemic" while the American Medical Association classify obesity as a disease. While we read that high BMI is becoming a very serious health issue, we need to be aware that not all those who have high BMI are unhealthy and those with "normal" BMI are healthy as recent studies in the US revealed that about 23.5% of "normal" weight adults have poor health while about half of the overweight adults are healthy. That is why it is important to go for medical screening so as to confirm our health status. Nonetheless, from the figure above, it is definitely better to have a "normal" BMI levels so one should still strive to have healthy BMI levels to reduce, not totally eliminate, poor medical health.

Chapter 2

Diet

One of the greatest pleasures in life is definitely eating. Yet, eating can also cause many problems to our health when it is not moderated. Most of us are aware that the basic guideline to a healthy diet is having three main meals with each meal being a balanced one. How we ascertain balance in a meal will be discussed later in this chapter. For most people being aware and adopting a balanced diet are two different things. A very busy worker who skips meal often and don't observe balanced portions in his meals will have his health deteriorate in the long run. In this chapter, we will look into these issues. Other topics that will be discussed include energy balance, weight loss/gain diet and how to fit in a healthy diet with minimal effort despite having a hectic schedule.

Energy Balance

Energy balance describes the state of equilibrium between how much we ingest (eat and drink) and how much we expand (physical activity). This balance is regulated automatically by our brain albeit biased towards an imbalance in favour of energy surplus (this will be discussed later). The diagram below can help explain the relationship between these determinants and its effects.

<u>Energy expenditure</u>
Daily physical activity/tasks and/or exercise

<u>Energy Intake</u>
Food and water

Weight maintenance
Energy Expenditure = Energy Intake

Weight Loss
Energy Expenditure > Energy Intake

Weight Gain
Energy Expenditure < Energy Intake

Whether we put on, lose or maintain our weight all depends on the understanding of the energy balance. Everything that we do, expend energy including sleeping. Almost everything that we put into our bodies by drinking and eating, is energy intake. The unit for energy is called kilocalories or kcal. Most of the time it is referred to simply as calories and used interchangeably.

Energy Expenditure

The total energy expended each day is made up of two components. The basal metabolic rate and the physical activity level. The former is the amount of energy used for basic functions of the human body like breathing, digesting, circulation of the blood etc, most of which we have no control over. So, it is correct to assume that even while sleeping or watching a movie at the cinema, we are actually burning calories. But very little. Basal metabolic rate differs from one person to another depending on age, gender and body weight. To find our basal metabolic rate, we can use a special weighing machine with electrical impedance capabilities. They are actually available quite widely and is quite affordable. To give an idea of the basal metabolic rate of a person, a 40 year old male of height 165m has a rate of around 1200 calories daily. Theoretically, if this person is in bed the whole day doing nothing, he would have to consume 1200 worth of food and water to maintain his or her weight. Anything more and he would gain weight and anything less, he would lose weight. There is only one thing that can influence basal metabolic rate and that is altering the amount of lean muscle mass in our body. The greater the amount of lean muscle mass, the higher is the rate and vice versa. To increase lean muscle mass, one would have to commit to a very intensive and structured weights training programme with a high protein diet. To reduce lean muscle mass, do nothing. As we age, we lose muscles. From the age of 25, our lean muscle loss is at a rate of 0.5% a year and this doubles to 1% as we enter the mid-30s. To defend muscle loss, regular weights training exercise 2 – 3 times a week would suffice. The other component of energy expenditure is physical activity and this itself is further divided into two. The first is functional and the other is discretionary. Functional physical activities refer to the things we do every day to survive like going to work, working, doing household chores, shopping etc. Of course the more physically demanding the job is, the greater is the energy expended. There are three categories; light, moderate and heavy. Light occupation refers to those jobs that use very little physical movement like desk bound jobs. On the other end of the spectrum, heavy occupation mostly refers to outdoor type jobs which require moving around and possibly carrying loads from point to point, like construction. Jobs like teaching and nursing fall in between under the moderate category. Discretionary physical activity quite simply refers to exercise. Exercise uses up the energy stored in our body and must be replaced at the end of the day otherwise a negative energy balance will occur. In the long run, this person will lose weight. The frequency, intensity, duration and type of exercise dictate the amount of calories burnt. This will be discussed in greater depth in Chapter 4 – Exercise.

The amount of energy we need each day is known as recommended daily allowance or RDA but I like to call it an energy budget. Just like how when we want to buy a house or a car, we have a budget, our daily energy intake also has a budget. Our daily energy budget depends on several factors, namely, age, gender, weight, type of occupation and level of physical activity. Below is a sample of my input. These options can be found at the HPB website.

- Age: 43
- Gender: Male
- Weight: 60
- Occupation
  - o Do not go to work.
  - o Have a light activity job, sitting most of the time e.g. office worker.
  - ✓ Have a moderate activity job with little time spent sitting down e.g. teacher, nurse or outdoor sales person.
  - o Have a heavy activity job e.g. construction or manual worker or a full-time sportsperson.
- Physical Activity Level
  - o Engage in light physical activities like walking slowly (strolling); mild stretching; sitting and playing with children; or light cleaning.
  - o Engage in moderate physical activities like walking briskly; slow leisure cycling; leisure swimming; mowing the lawn; ping pong; golf; tai chi; or heavy cleaning.
  - ✓ Engage in vigorous physical activities like climbing hills; aerobics; body building; jogging; or soccer, tennis, basketball, lap swimming or other competitive sports.

From the above input, my daily caloric budget is 2500 kcal. This means that this is the amount of calories that I must consume each day to maintain my weight. If I eat less than that, I will lose weight and if I eat more, I will gain weight. Similarly, if I exercise, I can lose weight and if I don't, I can gain weight. As mentioned before, by default, the human body is inclined to tip off the balance scale in favour of weight gain and the most common combination is a higher caloric diet with low or no physical exercise. That being said, effort to gain or lose weight must be deliberate and the attitude and motivation must be right.

Energy Intake

Whatever we consume will make up our energy intake. It is therefore very important to pay very close attention to what we consume. As the saying goes, "we are what we eat". Most of us eat three regular meals each day, breakfast, lunch and dinner. It is not wise to skip any meals as it would make one prone to snacking and binging which would eventually lead to gaining weight. But there is merit in breaking the portions of lunch and dinner into two smaller meals respectively. This would enable the body to have constant supply of energy throughout the day. I have met some health-conscious individuals who have five smaller meals a day as opposed to three main meals.

For our meals per se it is prudent to observe a balanced one. Recently, Health Promotion Board launched the My Healthy Plate approach as a guide towards healthy eating. The diagram can be seen below.

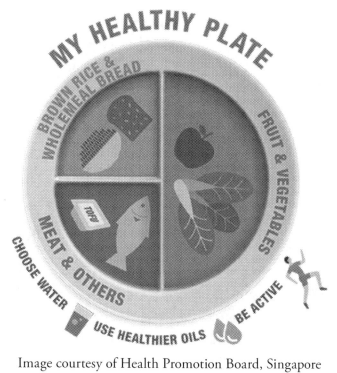

Image courtesy of Health Promotion Board, Singapore

This diagram gives a good idea of what a normal meal should consist of. The top right hand corner represents carbohydrates like rice, bread, noodles, potatoes, pasta etc. In this latest version, there is great emphasis on consuming wholegrain and moving away from refined grain products such as white bread, white rice and potatoes. This is because wholegrain products such as brown rice and wholemeal bread contains more fibre and nutrients and belongs to the low Glycemic Index or GI group. Taking food low in GI has several advantages. Firstly, it is digested slowly into the body thus making us feel full longer and therefore consuming less over time. This is a good way to lose weight. This group of food when consumed will also not cause a sudden increase in insulin in the blood. A spike in insulin into the blood stream helps to level the amount of carbohydrate in the bloodstream by converting it into fats and storing it slowly. If more frequent high GI food is consumed, the insulin may lose its effectiveness in performing their role and therefore will not be able to clear the glucose (the converted carbohydrate) in the bloodstream. The result is type 2 insulin resistant diabetes. And this process is irreversible. Low GI and hi GI food are also known as complex carbohydrate and simple carbohydrate respectively.

Food Preparation

Food preparation is another important factor to look into. There are many ways to prepare our food. The most common method of food preparation in our Asian kitchen involves boiling, stir frying, deep-frying, steaming, grilling, roasting, microwaving and more recently air-frying. To my knowledge, the healthiest way to prepare our food is by steaming as it is able to retain most of the original nutrients. Unfortunately, it is the least popular method of preparation. This is evident as our local chicken rice stalls usually offer more roasted chicken meat than steamed ones. Boiling, though as good as steaming as a way to prepare food, may result in the loss of some nutrients. However, not all is lost as these nutrients readily seeps into the water, so it is best to also consume the soup during the meals. Grilling or roasting is also a healthy choice of food preparation as it uses little or no oil at all. The use of microwave to prepare food has been controversial. Some has argued that nutrients in the food are reduced while others claim it can cause cancer. These claims have not been proven completely true which is why microwaves are still being sold in shops. My advice is, use it in moderation. While it is generally known that preparing food using oil is unhealthy, stir frying is generally acceptable, especially when used with healthier oils such as olive, canola and sunflower oil. Deep-frying is the unhealthiest though this method of cooking is the most popular. As it is the most versatile, over the years people have fried almost all types of food, not just meat. Vegetables and fruits have gone in that deep fryer. Food sellers have even perfected the art of frying ice cream. And as if frying food in its true form is not savory enough, flour have been added to increase its satisfaction, sometimes rendering the actual content of the food to just half.

For demonstration of this point, take a fried chicken wing from a fast food joint and separate the bone, meat and skin (with the flour) and you will discover that the amount of meat is actually quite meagre. Top of all food preparation which is the most nutritious is of course not preparing it at all, meaning, eating it raw, especially vegetables. For meat to be eaten raw, extra precaution has to be taken in terms of preparation. When we eat salads, we are eating the full potential of the nutritional content of the food. Nothing is lost as no heat is applied to the vegetables. The only problem with salad dishes is that it is usually eaten with dressing, which adds up the fat content and thereby increasing the caloric value of the food. In fact, a bowl of Caesar salad can contain more calories than a steak dinner. So if dressing has to be added in, choose the low fat version or even better, use the dressing my sister swears by, olive oil and lemon. But even if salad is eaten with dressing, I feel that it is even better than cooking it, in terms of nutritional value. In fact, it is my belief that salad is the saving grace of the Western diet. The reason why Caucasian BMI values for overweight starts at 25 and Asians at 23 is because of this. It may explain why a Caucasian of whose BMI value is 24 has less health problems than an Asian of similar value.

Processed Food

We have discussed the benefits of eating wholegrain over refined carbohydrates. In this paragraph, we will learn about the dangers of processed food. Quite simply, processed food refers to food that has other ingredients added to it. These other ingredients include oil, flour, sodium and preservatives. Because of the additives, it increases calories and fat content rendering it unhealthy. There are many processed food out there, the most popular being sausages. When I discovered sausages in my teens, I couldn't believe how cheap and delicious it was. I gobbled it down at every barbeque gathering I attended. It would appeal to all Singaporeans as it fits the formula of cheap and good. As I grew older, I learned that it was processed and embraced the wisdom of 'If it's too good to be true, then it probably is". Now I avoid it at all cost. Soon after that, I learn of other processed food such as crab sticks, sliced cheese, ham and nuggets. I am still discovering more as time goes by. An easy simple guideline to follow is to eat food in its true form. If chicken is the flavor of the day, then eat chicken, not the nuggets or sausages or ham versions. If fish is the one being craved, then get the real deal and not nuggets or fishballs.

Beverages

Believe it or not, beverages can also impact a good healthy nutritional plan in a negative way. Most beverages contain calories. A fizzy or gassy drink with 200 calories contains about 12 teaspoonfuls of sugar. Can you imagine pouring in 12 teaspoonful of sugar into your tea or coffee? Keep in mind that there are also calories in fruit juices. The ever popular bubble tea also contains calories that can add up to the daily caloric count. Drinks from coffee houses with fancy names and whip creams to add flavor or for aesthetic purposes also packs in the calories. Even sports drinks contain calories that would require us to run 10 – 15 minutes to burn it off. Today, some drinks from coffeeshops, food courts and hawker centres pack higher calories as they add on more ingredients into the commonly known beverages. In this case like Milo and Horlicks and adding prehistoric creatures titles onto their existing names to appeal to customers. All these beverages can easily add up to more than half of our Recommended Daily Allowance or RDA. In fact, for those people who takes in several sweetened drinks a day, losing weight can just be achieved by drinking plain water all day long. A good alternative to plain water which is flavoured and is gaining popularity among sports enthusiast today is coconut water. It has more potassium than banana, is real good at thirst quenching and almost fat free. If you're looking for beverages with zero calories, take comfort in knowing that coffee and tea are two of them, provided they are taken without milk and sugar. However, they are both diuretics, that is, they cause the body to rid itself of water. So make sure, water is taken to compensate the effect. Take precaution when drinking coffee with milk, especially with sweetened condensed and evaporated milk. Keep in mind that the type of milk mentioned is not actually real milk. They are made from hydrogenated palm oil, which is like pouring in oil into our favourite drinks like Teh Tarik. Be extra discreet when adding non-dairy creamer, mostly in powdered form, into the coffee and tea, they are also made up of vegetable fats which is high in saturated fats. They are present in most 2-in-1 and 3-in-1 coffee and tea sachets. Try to avoid them or at best limit its consumption.

Weight Loss

The American College of Sports Medicine or ACSM recommends daily caloric deficit of 500 - 1000 kcal daily to lose weight effectively. Why 1000kcal a day? Well, in one week this will amount to 7000 kcal which is almost equivalent to 1kg of body fats or in practical terms the loss of 1 kg body weight. Similarly, if 500 kcal is lost every day, one can lose about 0.5kg in body weight by the end of the week. In summary, 0.5 – 1kg weight loss is a good target to start with. Losing more than 1 kg per week is very difficult to maintain as I have observed in many of my students in the weight loss programme. Most usually end up gaining back the weight. This is because they probably had taken drastic actions to lose the weight. Such actions will add stress to the body and the mind and they usually would not want to have the same negative experience in the future. Furthermore, there is a limit as to how much fat can be used as an energy source in exercise and that is just 1kg weekly. If another source of energy is needed, the body will sacrifice the protein stores, which is literally our muscle and the depletion of muscle mass is counterproductive as it will lower the body's metabolic rate, which in turn will reduce the ability of the body to burn more calories. It is useful to know at this juncture that the use of fats and protein as energy sources is over and above the use of carbohydrate stores in the body.

On the other hand, losing less than 0.5 kg per week is not significant enough. Such difference in weight loss could just be due to removal of waste from the body and/or clothing. Similarly, small efforts to lose weight either through physical activity or diet will not result in significant weight loss. This is because, as part of its survival mechanism, the body is able to lower its metabolic rate to match the small differences in energy loss or deficit. For example, a brisk walk session of 20 minutes for a 90 kg person burns about 95 calories and one roti prata instead of the usual two saves 100 calories. These two examples given would hardly cause a dent in weight loss diet as the body compensate the loss in energy by lowering its metabolic rate. This explains why some people wonder why they are not losing weight despite the actions they had taken and the effort they have put in.

In his book, Fight the Fat, Dr Ben Tan recommends using a 40/60 rule of exercise and diet respectively. What he means is that 40% can be in the form of exercise and 60% loss can come from the diet. He has found this to be the most achievable and realistic combination. So, to lose 1000kcal each day, 400kcal should come from exercise and the 600kcal from food. For a 60kg person like me, to lose 400kcal I would have to run for almost one hour at a speed of 8km/hr, which is a slow jog speed. To lose 600kcal I can make simple substitutions. For example I can substitute coffee with milk (150 kcal), to black coffee (50 kcal) and save about <u>100 kcal</u>. In terms of snacks, instead of having an Old Chang Kee curry puff (360 kcal), I can substitute it with a fruit, for example a medium sized banana (105 kcal) and save <u>255 kcal</u>. For meals, I can choose more soupy dishes, especially the clear ones like prawn noodle soup (294 kcal). Eating that than a bowl of Mee Rebus (555 kcal) would save me another <u>226 kcal</u>. So, by just making simple modifications like these I actually reduce my caloric intake by 100 + 255 + 261 = 616 kcal. While these modification looks simple and easy to do and indeed, achievable in the first few days, to carry on this permanent change in lifestyle can be difficult. It requires determination, a strong motivation and resilience. We would be battling our inner urges as the energy balance is disrupted. These urges are primal and not to be underestimated. It is controlled by our subconscious mind which is more powerful and faster than our conscious mind. For this reason, weight modification is really a mental game. Strategies to overcome these urges will be discussed under the topic Mental Re-training. Dr Tan's formulae or approach corroborates with an article in the July 2013 edition of The ACSM Fit Society Page, a quarterly e-newsletter written for the general public. In it, exercise alone is reported not to be enough to lose weight.

Two issues of those among us who eat to their hearts content and never seem to gain weight and those who gained weight even though they have been doing the same thing and observe a similar diet over the years will be discussed in this paragraph. For the former issue, the reason why no weight increase is observed even though the person seems to be eating a lot is quite simple. This person has a high metabolic rate which is derived from the amount of lean muscle mass in the body. So whatever is eaten is burnt very quickly, so much so, there is no excess for the body to turn them into fats. Genetic disposition also dictates a more efficient way of using energy for everyday use. Also, observe the amount of food and type of food being eaten by these few 'lucky' individuals throughout the day or week. Chances are, the amount is small and they only eat 'big' meals once in a while. It is also inaccurate to assume that these people are healthy as some people with a small frame or doesn't appear to be overweight may still have higher fat content or cholesterol level as their body may store fats around the organs known as visceral fats, instead of under the skin or subcutaneous fats where it is more obvious. As for the latter case, where we find ourselves gaining weight even though no changes has been made to our diet or activity level, it is useful to note that our muscles actually starts shrinking as early as in our twenties. This condition is called Sarcopenia and has been discussed earlier. Recall that between the ages of 25 – 35, we lose 0.5% of our muscle mass each year and from age 35 onwards, we lose about 1% of our muscle mass. This means that our metabolic rate decreases which in turn means that our ability to burn calories, through the muscles, becomes less efficient and with that, the extra nutrients in our body is turned into fats.

Weight Gain

I have touched lightly on how to gain weight but perhaps it is a good time to emphasize in this section that weight gain is even harder to achieve than weight loss. As a PE teacher, I also look into the underweight students. Generally the level of success in achieving their target weight is even lower than their overweight counterparts. When dealing with weight gain, the greatest misconceived strategy is to eat as much 'junk' food as possible and be totally sedentary. This is quite reasonable to assume as it is the opposite strategy of losing weight. But adopting this strategy means the gaining of unhealthy weight. As mentioned before, gaining healthy weight is focused on gaining lean muscle mass. For this to happen, the subject has to consume lots of food high in protein and commit to a weights training regimen to bulk up. This form of weights training will be elaborated in Chapter 4 – Exercise. Food high in protein is not difficult to identify. They are found in many of the food we generally eat but to observe a high protein diet, one would have to consciously and conscientiously include it in every meal. King of all protein food and is considered the gold standard in protein content is the humble chicken egg. But most people avoid eating too many eggs because they are touted to be high in cholesterol. Recent evidences however point out that the cholesterol in eggs are not as damaging as what it was made out to be. Thus it is safe to introduce more eggs into the diet without increasing unhealthy cholesterol level in the body. Other high protein food includes tofu, cheese, tempeh, soya beans, nuts and seeds and milk. Some who are really serious take in protein powder or protein shake. I am not a fan of such unnatural product but I think it is safe enough to consume judging by the number of people who takes them.

The Amazing Human Thermostat

The human body has an internal regulator which helps the body to be in a state of homeostasis. Any lack of calories or negative energy balance will signal the central nervous system to stimulate our senses and the digestive system. When we feel hungry, our sense of smell will be keener, our eyes will be looking out for restaurant signboards and the ears will pick up the slightest sound of cooking. One particular nutrient will be on the top of the list, fats. So our noses will be looking out mostly fried stuff like Old Chang Kee delicacies etc. Why? Because fats is energy dense. 1kg of fats is equivalent to 9000 kcal as opposed to Carbohydrates, 4000 kcal and Protein, 4000 kcal. The prime directive from the brain is to get as much energy as possible for the body and quickly.

The Human Disposition:
The Famine that Never Arrived

Our body is in a constant state of energy acquisition and storage. This is part of the genetic predisposition of survival. As far as possible, it will horde energy in the body to the best of its ability. And by energy I mean food. The body is only able to store a relatively fixed amount of carbohydrates in the body, mostly in the muscles, liver and blood. Any extra carbohydrate ingested will be turned to fats. In terms of fats storage however, the body is capable of doing much better. Storage of fats in the body is infinite. The body is able to 'make adjustments' just so the body can store much more. The skin, for example, is able to stretch so as to accommodate the extra energy to be stored, which is usually under the skin anyway. For this argument, it is logical to conclude that an overweight person is the personification of a successful human design in terms of survivability. Survivability of what you may ask? Well, it is the survival of a famine, if ever there is one coming. An average human, is able to last between two to three weeks without food. However, an overweight person can last longer due to the excess energy stored in the form of fats under the skin. But most parts of the world famine is mostly rare or even if there is one, the world as a community has learned to overcome this natural calamity by helping one another through emergency supply efforts. Take note however that while the skin is able to adjust to increases in body weight, the skeletal system is not. Our bones and joints has been designed to only carry a certain amount of weight. Any excess will add additional stress to the joints especially. It is not surprising then that for most obese individuals, knee and back problems are rife. The most effective way to solve this problem rather than consulting medical practitioners is just simply reducing weight.

Conclusion

Eating in moderation should be the mantra of those who wish to lead a healthier lifestyle while nutrition and eating smart should be the action plan. In my earlier effort to lead a healthier lifestyle, I avoided my favourite group of food, Malay dishes, because I learn that most of the dishes are prepared with coconut milk and are often deep-fried. Later I became more discerning and learnt that I can still enjoy the dishes with some smart strategies like leaving the gravy out. Lontong is an example. It believe it is a complete balanced meal. The rice cake is carbohydrate, there's long beans, carrots, cabbage and turnip for vegetables. For protein, there's the powerful boiled egg and tofu. It is a power packed dish. Some Lontong dishes even have the great tempeh to boost the protein profile. The only misgiving is the gravy and coconut grating which are full of saturated fat. So I usually ask the makcik or vendor not to add the coconut grating or serunding and leave most of the gravy behind. Is it also possible to observe a healthy diet into a busy routine? Yes, with minimal preparation time and change in mindset. During weekdays, for example, I take my breakfast standing up in my kitchen as I gobble down my half boiled egg while preparing sandwiches for lunch for both me and my wife. I take about fifteen minutes to do these task which I consider an investment because during lunch, I save time travelling to the school canteen, buying food and sitting down to eat. I eat my sandwich at my cubicle answering emails or finishing up on lesson planning or writing reports. Plus I get to put healthy ingredients into my sandwiches. The fact that I have total control of what I put into my body give me great satisfaction. These simple modifications to the lifestyle can have significant and lasting positive effect on the quality of life.

Chapter 3

Rest

From knowledge and experience, this area is the first to suffer when work deadlines and assignments loom heavily over us. Lack of sleep or sleep deprivation has serious consequences to health and adequate sleep can improve the quality of our lives dramatically. Sleep, therefore, should be seen as an important and integral part of our daily routine. In this chapter, sleep related issues to be discussed will be; how many hours of sleep is considered adequate, what are the benefits of adequate sleep and vice versa, how to get good sleep, sleep debt, the power of napping and Circadian Rhythm.

Firstly, it is useful to understand the function of sleep. Scientists and researchers have long studied sleep and agree that one of the functions of sleep is consolidating what we have experienced and learned during the day. In fact, our learning is actively changed, restructured and strengthened during sleep. Memory is enhanced and stabilized while adequate sleep produces growth hormones necessary for building muscle mass and cell repair. Enough sleep has also been reported to increase hormones responsible for increasing resistance to common illnesses. Therefore sleep can enhance what we learn during the day be it learning a skill or acquiring knowledge.

On the other hand, sleep deprivation can be detrimental to health. It is reported that the amount of sleep we get is associated with mortality rate, that is, the more adequate sleep we get, the lower the mortality rate and vice versa. ACSM says that since sleep is necessary in regulating body processes, such as metabolism, the lack of it can lead to increase in appetite, energy deficit and weight gain as hormones are altered, especially cortisol, a stress hormones, which causes insulin in the body to be less resistant and thereby increasing the risk of diabetes. The Lancet, a medical journal, goes on further to assert that chronic sleep loss or insomnia increases the occurrences of diabetes, hypertension, obesity and memory loss. Symptoms of Insomnia include taking a long time to fall asleep, waking up many times at night, waking up early and unable to get back to sleep and waking up feeling tired most of the time. It is best to consult a doctor if symptoms such as these prevail over several weeks.

So how much sleep is adequate? It depends on many factors but generally, adult should get between 7-8 hours while school going children should get between 9 – 11 hours of sleep. For an adult to get 8 hours of sleep this means sleeping at 10pm and waking up at 6am. This seems like a reasonable timing unless of course there is a deadline the following day and the midnight oil lamp has to be lit. For school going children, the timing is harder to achieve. If they have to wake up at 6am to have 9hours of sleep so that they could use the bathroom and toilet, have breakfast and travel to school, this means that they would have to hit slumber land by 9pm and not many students I know sleep at 9pm. In fact, one of our keen observations as teachers is that some underperforming students usually get insufficient sleep. Underperformance is not only in the field of academic but also social and emotional development.

The term Circadian Rhythm will almost always turn up when discussing sleep. This is basically the biological clock that exist in all living things be it animals or plants or even micro bacteria. Understanding its characteristics may be advantageous. The sleep/wake cycle in humans is dependent on light and temperature. Thus it is natural to feel sleepy at night and awake in the morning. This is aided by the secretion of melatonin, a relaxing inducing hormone, at 9pm, which stops entering the blood stream at 7.30am. And what about dreams? Are they good? Well, according to studies, dream recall is mostly experienced by healthy individuals.

Havard Medical School has outlined a guide on how to get good sleep

- Avoid caffeine as they decreases the quality of sleep. These are found in coffee, tea, chocolate and cola. They should be consumed 4 – 6 hours before bedtime.
- The bedroom should be turned into a sleep-inducing environment. Soft, incandescent light, cool temperature, soft, slow music, heavy curtains, comfortable mattress will help create the mood to relax and sleep. If possible, work related assignments should not be done in the room especially on the bed. Pets that are active at night should be trained to only come to the room in the morning so that their owners can get complete rest.
- Establish a sleep routine like taking a bath 1 hour before sleeping. Others could be reading a book, watching TV or relaxation exercise. Strenuous exercise and discussing emotional issues should be avoided before sleeping.
- When waking up, if possible, natural lighting should be used. One way is to allow outside light into the room by drawing the curtains in the early morning.
- Go to bed and wake up the same time each day.
- Afternoon naps may be the culprit to poor sleep at night. If there is a need to nap, it should be short and before 5pm. Those who tend to take long afternoon naps for over an hour, some of them 2 – 3 hours and finding themselves hard to fall asleep at night. And when they do, it will be after midnight. When they wake up, they feel sluggish and make up by taking long naps in the afternoon again. The whole vicious cycle repeats itself.
- Eating before bedtime is unhealthy not because it will cause weight gain but because it will make sleep less restful as the digestive system

still has to work when it should be resting with the rest of the body system.

- Enough fluids should be drunk to prevent waking up at night thirsty or going to the toilet.
- If there is a need to exercise, it should be done at least 3 hours before sleep.

But what if, with all these measures, the right amount of sleep is still unable to be achieved? Scientific American online calls this situation, 'sleep debt' or the difference between the amount of sleep one should be getting and the amount of sleep one actually gets. According to the website, the body will have to make up for 'lost' hours of sleep on other days and occasions. Perhaps a couple of extra hours in bed over the weekend for sleeping late on a weekday night preparing for an important presentation. Whatever it is, it has to be repaid, highlighting that it is foolish to think that one can train oneself to be a 'short sleeper'. The effect of long term or chronic sleep debt is the same as what was discussed earlier, that it can lead to obesity, insulin resistance (diabetes) and heart disease, on top of a condition where the brain gets foggy, vision is impaired and memory is negatively affected.

Everyone has experienced the positive effect of a short afternoon nap. Thus, it should not be surprising when WebMD reports that a 15 – 20 minute nap can increase alertness and improve motor function. In addition, napping has also been associated with boosting the memory, cognitive skills and creativity, reduce stress and even decrease the risk of heart disease. Napping is touted to be better than coffee in increasing alertness level overall. As a guide, napping should be consistent with a schedule best between the hours of 1pm – 3pm. It should also be less than 30 minutes. Working at the office, slumping on the office chair or resting the head on the desk are good, discreet positions just as long as it is comfortable. A soft, small pillow can do wonders to the quality of the nap.

As discussed above, resting is a crucial part of health which can affect our physical, social and mental development. It is unfortunate that resting has not been given its due importance in our society. It is the first casualty of a busy schedule for most adults and it is mostly taken for granted by students due to the lack of understanding. So far, issues pertaining to sleep are mostly attributed to sleep deprivation and many studies have been launched to study its effects and causes.

Chapter 4

Exercise

This chapter will be the most thorough in the book. To me, exercise is the most important component of health. It is the key to improving the other components and some of its benefits cannot be derived elsewhere. For example, both exercise and a healthy diet are effective ways one can approach in managing weight but diet alone will not be able to increase muscle mass or improve cardio respiratory function. Other areas exercise can develop that dieting alone cannot is in the social and mental domain. For example, playing team sports helps increase social network while mental development is achieved when strategizing games tactics or analyzing skill technique. Exercise also produces the natural 'feel good' drug in the body called endorphins which helps us manage stress and gives us the drive to work or play harder. In this chapter you can look forward to learning about,

- the definition of exercise,
- exercise recommendations,
- exercise for fitness: FITT & Training Principles,
- exercise for weight control.

The Definition of Exercise: Physical Well-being

According to the WHO, Physical well-being refers to a state where all the body system work well with no injuries and illnesses. The body is also able to carry out every day physical tasks. Today, however, it is not always easy to achieve a state of physical well-being, let alone retain or maintain one's overall state of health. Many of us are able to carry out every day physical tasks but how many of us are able to claim we are free of injuries and illnesses. Several years back I was told that my cholesterol level was high and when I related this to a friend of mine, he said that it was normal to have that in Singapore. While it gave me a sense of comfort hearing that, I was alarmed at the state of mind of people today where it has become a normalcy and acceptance to have high cholesterol level. Are we okay with living our lives taking medication every day or seeing the doctor every few months just to sustain our current lifestyle? That is really something that we all have to seriously ask ourselves. For those of us who meet the definition of physical well-being by WHO, the challenge is to maintain it and for those who are not, the ensuing sections will help achieve it.

Exercise Recommendation also known as Physical Activity Guidelines

What does exercise recommendations entail? If these recommendations were carried out, the one doing it would most likely able to be physically healthy and avoid contracting lifestyle diseases. Exercise recommendations, or sometimes called, prescriptions or guidelines, are revamped every several years where this is done to adjust to changes in trends, most often than not, an unhealthy one. Usually, the latest recommendations are the most comprehensive and customized.

In the second half of 2011, HPB launched the National Physical Activity Guideline for adults and older adults. A couple of years later, guidelines for children and youth were released. These guidelines were intended to inform stakeholders about the relationship between lifestyle and health. Four groups of people were identified and for each group, four dedicated exercise recommendation were issued. The guidelines is replicated below

<u>Young children (below 7 years)</u>
Aerobic Activity

- For infants, physical activity should be encouraged from birth, particularly through floor-based play in safe environments.
- Children capable of walking unaided should be physically active (structured and unstructured) for at least 180 minutes spread throughout each day in safe environment.

Sedentary Behaviour

- Limit total sedentary entertainment screen time (e.g. television and video games) to <2 hours per day.

<u>Children and Youth (7 to 18 years old)</u>
Aerobic and Strength Activity

- Accumulate 60 minutes or more of moderate to vigorous intensity physical activity every day, emphasizing aerobic type physical activities.
- Incorporate vigorous intensity physical activity (including those that strengthen muscles and bones) on at least 3 times a week as part of the 60 minutes

Sedentary Behaviour

- Limit total sedentary entertainment screen time (e.g. television and video games) to < 2 hours per day.
- Break up sedentary periods (except time spent sleeping) lasting longer than 90 minutes with 5 to 10 minutes of standing, moving around, active play, or doing some physical activity.

For children and youth, 60 minutes of activity time each day seem to be quite difficult to achieve. A recent study by professor Michael Chia of the National Institute of Education reported that none of the 244 secondary school students involved in the study was able to achieve the national guideline of one hour physical activity daily. This is actually worrying as these youth will potentially become unhealthy adults. For the first time, the guidelines have included recommendations on sedentary behavior which I think is really interesting and wonderful. I would think it is because of the advent of hand phones and computers. I have seen how these gadgets have 'taken control' of my own children and how they have negatively impacted some of my students' school life. Initially, my wife and I thought that our children should have or do what the Jonses have or do, so that when their friends talked about it, they are not left out. Soon after, our TV gets connected to the X-box game console, our computers had games icons on its screen, their laps was littered with Sony PSP, Nintendo DS and Apple i-pads. Our older children are smartphone equipped. At first, monitoring was minimal but soon we realized that they became less active and even affected their behavior for example they were slow to react to instructions. There were even occasions when they exhibited unruly and rowdy behavior. That became unacceptable. So, we introduced restrictions and boundaries. But it was, and still is, very difficult to enforce the two-hour screen time guideline. Restricting their screen time essentially meant that, we as parents, have to fill the void. This is especially difficult as we always look forward to the weekend to wind down after a hectic work week and as soon as we give them their 'alone time' so we can put our feet up, they would engage themselves with the screens. To be honest, we are still looking for more effective ways to manage the situation.

Adult (19 to 49 years old)
Aerobic

- Accumulate 150 minutes of moderate-intensity or 75 minutes of vigorous-intensity aerobic activity per week. Individuals can combine vigorous intensity and moderate-intensity activities, with 1 minute of vigorous-intensity aerobic activity being equivalent to 2 minutes of moderate-intensity aerobic activity. Aerobic activity should be performed for at least 10 minutes per session. Combinations of moderate intensity and vigorous-intensity aerobic activities can be performed to meet this recommendation.

Strength

- Strength activities provide additional health benefits. These include muscle-, bone- and joint-strengthening activities (e.g. using handheld weights, resistance bands, calisthenics, strength-training equipment, dragon boating, and rock climbing) and some mind-body exercises (e.g. *Qigong, Tai Chi*, Yoga and Pilates). Strength activities should involve major muscle groups: legs, hips, back, abdomen, chest, shoulders and arms.

Adult (50+ years old)
Aerobic Activity

- To acquire substantial health benefits, adults need to accumulate 150 minutes of moderate-intensity or 75 minutes of vigorous-intensity aerobic activity per week. Individuals can combine vigorous-intensity and moderate-intensity activities, with 1 minute of vigorous-intensity aerobic activity being equivalent to 2 minutes of moderate-intensity aerobic activity. Aerobic activity should be performed for at least 10 minutes per session. Combinations of moderate intensity and vigorous-intensity aerobic activities can be performed to meet this recommendation.

Strength Activity

- Strength activities provide additional health benefits. These include muscle-, bone- and joint-strengthening activities (e.g. using hand-held weights, resistance bands, calisthenics, strength-training equipment, carrying groceries and climbing the stairs) and some mind body exercises (e.g. Qigong, Tai Chi, yoga and Pilates). Strength activities should involve major muscle groups: legs, hips, back, abdomen, chest, shoulders and arms.

Balance

- In addition, balance ability may become a concern for some older adults as they age. Balance is maintained or improved by regularly following the physical activity guidelines for older adults.

The most noticeable change in the new exercise guideline is the amount of time allocated. 150 minutes may seem such a big amount but essentially it is quite the same as the old guideline. If the 150 minutes were broken down, it would basically mean 5 times of half an hour, each time. The component that is totally new is the inclusion of strength training into the guideline. This makes a lot of sense as, as mentioned before, our lean muscle starts to shrink in our mid 20s and accelerates 10 years later. A drop in lean muscle mass invites a whole lot of problem as the metabolic rate decreases. Strength training thus serves to defend this muscle loss and is not meant to actually increase it, although it is not such bad thing when that happens. Strength training is even more important as we approach our golden years. That is when our bones starts to degenerate and affect the structural integrity of our body. Aerobic exercises such as swimming and cycling does little to increase bone health. Running helps but too much of it can cause the joints to weaken especially the knee. For teachers coming out of retirement, getting involved in activities like yoga and taichi is recommended to increase a greater sense of balance as one of the major causes of death in Singapore is medical condition related to falls. Whatever it is, getting enough exercise is a major challenge for adults. Most studies show that young adults are relatively active until they start working and the amount of exercise gets cut even further as they set up families. Then, as poor health condition and illnesses sets in, most of the time into the thirties, some will start to exercise while a good majority continues with the largely sedentary lifestyle and poor diet. The findings also point out that women are less active than men and that career and family seem to be the main stumbling block to getting enough exercise. So the very first thing that needs to be addressed is managing time to exercise. This will be discussed in Chapter 7.

Exercise for Fitness

Exercise should be an integral part of our effort to be physically healthy and to ensure that we function at an optimal level physiologically. Having enough exercise has many benefits and the lack of exercise has many disadvantages. How to exercise seems to be the most common question so I shall try to provide some guidelines. If you are the sort that likes structure, like me, then carry on reading but if you are the type that are more intuitive, like my wife, then you can skip this section. Both have their merits but like I always tell my students and children, "If you fail to plan, you plan to fail." Essentially, there are two types of principles; one is for the beginner or novice – the FITT Principle and a more advance one for the avid or serious fitness junkie – Principles of Training.

The FITT Principle

FITT stands for F – Frequency, I – Intensity, T – Type, T – Time.

Frequency

This means how many times a week to exercise. Both HPB and ACSM has de-emphasized this component of the principle. The number of times to exercise in a week now is dependent on the total accumulated hours per week. For example, adults between the ages of 19 to 49 years old are to accumulate 75 minutes of vigorous intensity aerobic activity per week. This could mean 25 minutes 3x/wk or 15 minutes 5x/wk. Technically, one could also do a vigorous 75 minute workout one day and rest for the next six days but I personally feel spreading out the duration to get more frequency to be better. This is generally for aerobic exercises. For resistance training HPB recommends doing it twice a week while ACSM, two to three times weekly.

Intensity

Intensity refers to how hard we exercise. There are several ways to determine this, the commonest is by measuring our heart rate during exercise. We can do this by placing the tip of our fore and middle finger over the underside of where the lower arm meets the wrist. The pulse can be felt at the upper half, nearer to the thumb. We would need a watch to determine the heart rate per minute accurately. Count the number of times the pulse beat over 15 seconds and then multiply by 4. This will give us the heart rate per minute. But what does this all mean? Well, how hard we exercise will determine not only the training effect but also the type of energy stores used for the exercise. But before we can explore this interesting topic, we need to first determine our maximum heart rate or MHR. This can be determined by subtracting our age from the number 220. That is, if I am 40 years old, my MHR would be 220 – 40, which is 180 beats per minute or BPM. To exercise effectively, we need to exercise at a percentage of the MHR and is usually within zones. For example, after a few rounds the track I took my heart rate and recorded 126 BPM. This is equivalent to 70% of my MHR. At this intensity I am actually using an equivalent amount of carbohydrate and fats to sustain my physical activity. My cardio vascular endurance or aerobic capacity will also somewhat improve. Any harder and I will use less fats and more carbohydrate and improvement to my aerobic endurance will be greater, vice versa. What about other intensities? The exercise heart rate zone below is taken from Timex Digital Heart Rate Monitor Guide.

Zone	Percent (%)	Level	Purpose
5	90% - 100%	Very Hard	Improvement in speed as aerobic and anaerobic capacity increases
4	80% - 89%	Hard	Significant improvement to aerobic capacity
3	70% - 79%	Comfortably Hard	Cardiovascular improvement and moderate improvement to fitness
2	60% - 69%	Moderate	Some improvement to fitness. Good for burning fats
1	50% - 59%	Easy	General maintenance of health with little or no improvements

By now you should be wondering about how hard to calculate heart rate during exercise and how intrusive it is to do so. Luckily, many watch and sports companies have invented something called the heart rate monitor or HRM. They come in many shapes and sizes but the most common is the use of a chest strap sensor which is placed just under the sternum. It will communicate with the accompanying watch and can give us instantaneous feedback, that is, the watch will display at what percentage or the actual heart rate we are exercising in. More expensive models will allow us to set the heart rate zones according to our training or exercise needs. For example, we can set the watch at zone 3 and carry on with our activity like running. When our heart rate falls below 70% the watch will beep to indicate that we are exercising below the targeted exercise heart rate. To eliminate the beeping, we will have to increase intensity by running faster. A different beep will indicate going over 80% or we are running too fast. Again, we have to slow down. Such devices are very convenient and help to achieve our goals more effectively. To be more effective in our training is to determine first what intensity our workout will be rather than just working out and then determine at what intensity the workout was at. Usually, it is prudent to have a mix of different intensities in our training. For example, if we schedule three workouts in a week, one should be in Zone 3 where we can go longer distance or duration, another one should be in Zone 4 or 5 where we most likely will be doing fartlek training or intervals for shorter duration and distance and another at Zone 1 or 2 for recovery and general maintenance. The use of a heart rate monitor is convenient but it has its own limitations for example, anxiety can increase the heart rate artificially which will make the reading inaccurate. I also discovered that medication can increase heart rate too. There are other ways to determine intensity, one being the use of RPE or Rate of Perceived Exhaustion sometimes known as the Borg Scale. This does not require any equipment, just our own perception of how hard the exercise or training is.

RPE Level	HR%	Level	Benefit	With company	Alone
1-2	50 – 60%	Easy	Recovery & General maintenance	Can hold a conversation easily	Breathing is easy like normal. Can do complex mental division and multiplication.
3-4	60 – 70%	Moderate	Fat burning benefit	Can hold a conversation with some effort	Breathing is slightly harder. Can do simple mental multiplication and division.
5-6	70 – 80%	Comfortably hard	Aerobic improvement	Takes effort to hold a conversation	Breathing is harder. Can do mental addition and subtraction.
7-8	80 – 90%	Hard	Fitness building – Optimalfitness building	Can give short responses only	Breathing is hard. Can do simple mental addition and subtraction.
9-10	90 – 100%	Very Hard	Anaerobic improvement for speed	Cannot talk	Out of breath. Cannot do any form of mental calculations.

The table above shows how heart rate can correspond with our RPE. The description in working out with company or alone is something I experienced and may vary from one to another.

Some experts have cited RPE to be better in determining exercise intensity over the use of HRMs and I couldn't agree more. The only problem I faced was recording it down as HRM automatically keeps a log of our workout dates and level of intensities. So the use of RPE should be accompanied with manual recordings. Also remember to determine first what intensity our workout should be at before starting rather than vice versa. Be aware too that there are other more detailed and accurate ways to measure exercise intensity which are usually very costly and more for the professional athletes.

<u>Type</u>

This refers to the type of exercise that we can engage ourselves in. The exercise that we mostly engage in is called aerobic or endurance exercise, a type of cardio-vascular or cardio-respiratory exercise. This involves running, swimming, cycling, skipping, aerobics, sports such as football, basketball, badminton and so on. Those who go to the gym and carry weights involve themselves in resistance or strength training although it can be done by using our own body weight such as doing pushups and pull ups. Yoga, *Tai Chi, Qigong* and Pilates are types of mind body exercises or MBE and they are responsible for improving our strength, flexibility and balance.

Aerobic exercise must be the staple of our exercise buffet because it offers the most benefit to the daily functioning of internal body system. With these types of exercises, lifestyle diseases such as high blood pressure, stroke, some types of cancer, heart disease can be prevented or managed or even improved. This type of exercise should also be on the top list of those who wants to lose weight. This is because aerobic activities done at the right intensity and duration can directly tap on the fats for energy. For example, exercising between 60 – 70% of our HRmax will roughly use 50% of energy from fats. I would say, that MBE exercises are not very effective for weight loss. They have a different purpose as mentioned above.

When I discovered about my poor health and wanted to lose weight, I researched on the most effective and safe way to achieve my objective and discovered the sports of triathlon. Many people have misconceptions about this sport. The most common reaction is that it's very tough and the second most common reaction is that it's dangerous. It is actually far from these two misconceptions. Triathlon consists of three activities executed one after another; swimming, cycling and running. Running alone is a very dangerous activity because the constant pounding on the ground will eventually injure the knee unless measures are taken like running on soft surfaces and knee strengthening exercises are done regularly. This is why running has been categorized as a high impact activity. Swimming and cycling however offer similar aerobic benefits with very much less negative effect on the knee joint. These three activities executed together will also develop the overall musculature of the human body. While running develops the hamstring and gastrocnemius (calf) muscles, cycling works mainly on the quadriceps and swimming targets the upper body. This will result in a balanced muscular growth while still improving the cardio vascular system. As triathlon has three sports in one, weekly training will hardy consist of more than two of the same activity. In fact, we can just do one of each and we can be ready for our first triathlon called a mini-triathlon. This consists of a 200 meters swim in the open sea, which is equivalent to about 4 laps of an Olympic sized pool. The cycling part is just a mere 10km which should take an average person about 30 minutes to complete. After coming down from the bike, participants complete a short 2km run. In total it would take less than an hour. I think that's a lot more interesting than running 10km which takes about the same time.

However effective aerobic exercise can benefit the human body, certain physical development or improvement cannot be achieved by just doing aerobic based activities as mentioned above. That is why strength training has been included in the exercise guidelines albeit just recently. The reason is strength training have specific benefits aerobic exercise cannot achieve. Strength training is also very effective for managing weight gain as it helps increase the body's metabolic rate by increasing lean muscle mass.

ACSM recommends adults to perform two to four sets of exercise on each muscle group. For each set, execute 8 – 12 repetitions to improve strength and power, 10 – 15 repetitions to improve strength in middle age and older persons starting exercise and 15 – 20 repetitions to improve muscular endurance. What does all these mean? Repetitions refers to the number of times an exercise is performed. For example, if we do 10 push-ups, then that's 10 repetitions or reps. 1 set means that the exercise was performed for 1 round, like at the end of the 10 push-ups, it is counted as 1 set. If another 10 push-ups is done, then 2 sets have been performed. This is mostly how people train in the gym. The major muscle groups in the body mentioned before refers to big muscle groups. Below are the names of the muscle groups and the type of exercises that can be done at the gym to train them. Look them up on *Youtube* to see how each exercise is performed.

1. Biceps – Bicep Curls
2. Triceps – Triceps Extensions
3. Pectorals – Chest Press
4. Latissimus Dorsi – Lats Pull
5. Abdominals – Sit Ups
6. Quadriceps – Leg Press
7. Hamstring – Hamstring Curls
8. Gastrocnemius – Calf Extension

These are quite complete and specific resistance training exercises. But for most of us, going to the gym is not realistic as it can be time consuming and costly. I have developed a type of resistance training exercise which can be done at the comfort of our own home and use just our own body weight. Furthermore it is quick, just in 30 minutes. I call it the Pyramid 100. It has been modified from the US Marines Training Manual. The exercises are

1. Push-ups
2. Sit ups
3. Lunges
4. Single Leg Calf Raises

Instructions

1. Follow the following sets and reps for each exercise

    i. Set 1: 18 Reps
    ii. Set 2: 20 Reps
    iii. Set 3: 24 Reps
    iv. Set 4; 20 Reps
    v. Set 5: 18 Reps
    Total: 100 Reps

2. Have only 30 seconds between exercises and about 2 minutes between sets.
3. It doesn't matter how the exercise is performed, the reps should try to be observed so that one will have the feeling of accomplishment of completing 100 reps at the end of the session. For example, instead of a full sit up, crunches can be performed.

As can be seen, the exercise is called a pyramid because the repetition goes up from the beginning and peaked at set 3 after which it declines in repetitions. I usually perform the Pyramid 100 in front of the TV while watching the news. The 30 minutes slot is just nice for me to watch the news at 9.30pm.

Working out in groups or individually is also another factor to consider. As discussed earlier, experts assert that group workouts can ensure greater continuity when members depend on each other. However, working out in groups also has its drawbacks. When the planned session is cancelled due to unforeseen circumstances, there is a high chance that the activity would also be put off. For example, when one of my Saturday morning group ride is cancelled due to the weather or other factors, most of us would take the opportunity to stay in bed. The motivation to get out of bed to exercise on our own is just not strong enough. For this reason, I would recommend adopting a dual mode of exercise, group and individual. This is especially so for those who were games players in the past. Former team players like football, basketball, badminton and so on usually are able to meet during the weekends to play. This is due to work and family commitments. However, the frequency and duration is too low for the body to be healthy. These weekend games workout must be supplemented by weekday individual exercise which is easily attainable by going for a brisk walk, jog, swim, gym work or spin on a bike. There is no need to wait for one another.

Time
<u>Time</u>

The amount of time recommended is, as discussed, 150 min of moderate intensity or 70 minutess of vigorous intensity exercise. For both durations, aerobic activity is preferred. At first glance 150 minutes look intimidating and unachievable but if it is broken down it looks really easy. For example, if 150 minutes is broken down into 5 days, so that we can work out from Monday to Friday, that would mean just 30 minutes a days. That 30 minutes can be further broken down into 2 sessions, before and after work. One of the safest exercise to do other than swimming and highly recommended for those whose BMI is 27.5 and above or those with knee problems is brisk walking. This exercise is especially convenient for those whose main transport to work is about 15-20 minutes walk away from home. For example, skip the feeder bus and walk to and from the MRT station. But remember, the walk has to be brisk enough to break us into a light sweat, so it's convenient to bring a small towel. There are many possible combinations we can do to meet the recommended 150 or 75 minutes of exercise and the best to me is when it is customized to our daily lifestyle. For example, incorporating these exercises into our daily routines is highly possible to achieve where one can commit before and after work, not to mention during one's commute to and fro destinations. Sometimes, special planning has to be done to ensure little or no disruption to daily life. For example, having a spare set of work clothes in the office or having a set of wet gear in the car in case there is time after work for some laps in the pool.

Do remember that under the guideline, two sessions of strength training also have to be done weekly to ensure that muscular, joint and bone strength are looked into. Again, try incorporating it into our daily routine. Personally, I find it hard to bring myself to the gym so I usually do my pyramid 100 at home, in my air-con room while watching the tv. The time taken is just about right, I don't have to leave the house and my family is still by my side.

How about exercising more than the recommended guideline? This would mean going against the adage, 'Too much of a good thing is a bad thing'. Is this necessarily so? For example, professional athletes and enthusiast can train up to 10 times a week, taking a day off one of the week days and exerting themselves twice a day on some days. Each training can take up to several hours. It is important that we know that this is achieved after years of dedicated training and is done progressively. This is possible because the human body is highly adaptable but again this is not for everybody. In determining the duration of exercise we should know our limits. I would deem it prudent to look at how much energy our body can support our activity. In our body, we use mainly two forms of fuel, carbohydrate and fats. While carbohydrate is the preferred fuel, fats utilization for physicals activity is also actively used but sparingly. They are used in different amount depending on the intensity of the exercise, the harder the workout, the more carbohydrates are used and the less fats are mobilized and vice versa. Carbohydrate storage in the form of glycogen is also much smaller than fats therefore being able to fuel the body for only a moderate amount of time, approximately 90 to 120 minutes of moderate intensity exercise. Once glycogen stores are depleted, the person may experience a negative situation called 'bonking' which is a feeling of extreme physical exhaustion and light headedness. Beyond this point, if physical activity continues the main fuel will almost solely will come from fats but because fat conversion to glycogen is a longer and slower process, the subject has to slow down or the body may have to shut down and this can be very dangerous. 90 to 120 minutes of exercise can fuel a run from 10 to 21km, cycle from 40 to 60 km, swim for about 60 laps and play a full basketball, football or badminton game. For that, I would recommend that we should limit ourselves to these distances and duration. Having said that, we can and should also pursue our aspiration to attempt longer distances like the 42km Marathon race. However preparations must be taken seriously to prepare our body to run continuously between 4 to 6 hours for beginners.

The Principles of Training

Principles of training is a guide most athletes, serious or enthusiasts use to improve their performance. There are about four major principles.

1. Specificity,
2. Overload
3. Progression
4. Reversibility

Specificity

The type of training we do should be as close as possible to the sports or physical activity that we want to improve. For example, if we want to improve our 2.4km run for IPPT or NAPFA, then our training should consist mainly running. While this is quite common sense others may still make wrong assumptions. For example, some people may cycle to improve their running time. While cycling will improve the cardio respiratory system, which will be the main contributor for the run, it will lack in the effect of improving the muscles needed for a run. With that in mind, games players such as basketball and football, may not benefit much from a long continuous run as they do not do so during a game. They would benefit more greatly if they adopt interval training. Even the time of day matters when dealing with specificity. I remember feeling very taxed during a race where I had to cycle, by that time, about 11am. The hot afternoon soon took a toll on the cycling portion of the event because most of my training was done in the early morning. A friend then told me that I should include cycling in the afternoon as part of my training. While specificity is a very important principle, it is not wrong to adopt some variety into our training, especially to avoid injury and even more so for mental reasons because just doing one sports can be monotonous over time. So it is quite alright to throw in a swim or a spin here and there when training for a marathon.

Overload

For improvement, training should also adopt the principle of overload where the training load is more than the actual activity. Overload can take on many forms. It can be in terms of duration or load in weight. For example, when training for a 10km run, one or two of the training run distance should be longer than the actual race distance ranging anything between 12 to 15km. Ankle weight is another example of using the principle of overweight where when used, will make the person put in the extra effort to move so that on the actual day of performance or competition will feel lighter. However, putting on extra weight to the body can cause additional stress to the joints and bones and should be used only with the advice of fitness professionals. Another way to overload the cardio respiratory system is to increase intensity. This can be in the form of interval and fartlek where the body is subjected to harder effort, more than the actual run itself. Intervals and fartleks can be done in almost all discipline including, running, swimming and cycling. Team sports such as basketball, football, badminton, softball also can benefit from these two training methods. As long as the workout is harder than the actual performance, it can be deemed using the system of overload. This principle is important as it will enable the body not to feel so taxed on the actual race day because it had done worse before. In fact many fitness enthusiasts will tell you that it is a short cut to increased performance.

<u>Progression</u>

This principle looks into how training load or volume should be increased regularly to bring about increased performance. The human body is highly adaptable to changes. For example, if we exercise for 30 minutes, 3 times a week, each day for a month, we will experience a drop in improvement after several weeks of the same workout. In other words, the greatest noticeable improvement one can feel is at the beginning of the workout. Thus it is important that we increase the training volume on a weekly basis. But what does it mean by volume? It could mean distance or time. For example if we track the amount of our exercise by the distance, total up the weekly distance or mileage like if Monday we ran for 5km, Thursday, 3 km and Sunday, 8km, then the weekly mileage is 16km. Or if Monday run took us 30 minutes and Thursday and Sunday run was 20 minutes and 1 hour respectively, then the total exercise time for the week is 1 hour and 50 minutes. As a rule of thumb, most exercise enthusiast and athletes increase their load between 10 – 15%. Thus in the example above, the following week's training mileage should be around 18km or 2 hours and 5 minutes. Athletes and serious enthusiasts adopt a training system of progression called sports periodization. There are 3 components namely macrocycle, mircocycle and mesocycle. The biggest component is called the macrocycle. This takes a year and centers around the main competition or race for example training for a full marathon at the Standard Chartered Singapore Marathon. Planning is done so much so that the athlete will peak at the event. Within this period there are three phases called preparation, competitive and transition. Briefly, the preparation stage is where we build our aerobic base, learn about techniques, strategies or rules of the competition or game. At the competition stage, training is ramped up and we may take on several smaller competitions leading up to the main one. The transition stage is a post-race period where we relax and involve ourselves in light, recreational training. As mentioned, training for a full 42km marathon may take up to a year. Even that, we should have already been able to run 10km comfortably and have attempted a few half marathons. That being said, the transition stage starts in December after the event. This may take up till March or April. The preparation phase follows, lasting 3 to 4 months all the way up to August. The competition phase kicks in next where we should have signed up for a couple of 10 to 15km runs. The following months we should attempt 21km half marathons. The Army Half Marathon, a running event organized by the Singapore Armed Forces usually held in September, is an excellent opportunity to test one's fitness in running a half marathon. Another running event called the Newton Challenge which is usually held in October, gives runners the opportunity to attempt a longer distance of 32km. If executed correctly, we should be able to peak by the main event itself. The Microcycle refers to just a week of training. The focus is the frequency, type, duration, distance and intensity of training done during that week. This can range from 3 times a week to up to 10, depending on how serious we are and what kind of performance we want to achieve. The type of exercise is important to elicit maximum training effect. Typically we should include at least one speed (eg intervals), one strength (fartlek) and one endurance training (long continuous easy run). Strength and flexibility training such as resistance training and/or pilates and yoga can also prove useful for overall development. It is important put aside at least one day of the week with no activity for the body to rest. Usually the total distance or duration of the run or exercise is totaled up weekly so as to ascertain at which point of the Macrocycle we are at. The Mesocycle is the last component we will discuss. Mesocycle looks at a group of microcycle from 2 – 6 weeks. For example a Mesocycle with a group of 4 Microcyle will last about a month and will observe 3 weeks of continual progression with 1 week of recovery phase. For example if the weekly mileage for week 1 in the preparatory stage of the Macrocycle training for a marathon, is 20km, week 2 should be 22km and week 3 can be 25km but the week 4 weekly mileage can drop back to 22km. At the start of the next Mesocycle, week 1 weekly mileage can pick up again at 25km, peaking at 30km in week 3 before dropping back down to 28km in week 4. This goes on until at the peak of the competition phase of the Macrocycle, we should be clocking a weekly mileage of 84km with a long run lasting at least 35km. This is no easy feat and as we can imagine it takes a lot of discipline, will power and very skillful time management. Truthfully, I was never able to attain such a high weekly mileage in training in both my marathons that I attempted because of my busy work schedule and my responsibilities as a father. A long weekend run of 30 km and above would mean running for at least 3 over hours and this does not include preparation and recovery which would eventually take almost the whole day leaving me unable to interact with my family. Because of that, I decided that marathon is not for me at this point in my life. Perhaps I will attempt to do this once my children have grown up.

Reversibility

With reversibility, we basically would lose the training effect after a period of time. Textbook placed this duration as 2 weeks but enthusiast often would feel that they get sluggish as soon as just a few days. What this principle mean is that we have to train continually or regularly otherwise we will lose all that hard work.

Exercise for Weight Management

While it is possible to control our weight without exercise, ie, by dieting alone, this is not recommended because exercise has its own unique advantages of which dieting cannot achieve. This includes optimal muscular function which will result in greater strength, muscular endurance and flexibility. This cannot be achieved by just ingesting protein. With weight bearing exercises like resistance training, exercise will make the bones stronger. This also cannot be achieved with just ensuring calcium rich food gets in the diet. With cardio exercises too, the circulatory and respiratory system will improve to enable the individual to complete his or her daily task with great proficiency and without feeling breathless or tired. And this cannot be achieved with just eating good carbohydrates like whole grain bread or brown rice.

Exercise for Weight Loss
Aerobic activity

- HPB recommends a duration of 150 to 250 of moderate intensity aerobic exercise with some maybe needing to do more than that. It states that a caloric imbalance of minimum 500kcal daily is needed to lose 0.5kg per week. This by no means an easy task. To lose 500 calories one would need to run about 5 miles or 8km each day. That is why it is more practical to combine it with reduction in input.

Strength Training

- This is also important to build lean muscle mass which will in turn increase the metabolic rate of the body.

It is important that we understand how our body works. Firstly the human body was optimally designed for survival. Its main aim is to horde the most efficient fuel into the body, fats, and convert any other excess substrate like

72

sugar, glucose or carbohydrate into fats (1kg of fats=7700kcal vs 1kg glucose = 4400kcal). The body does two other things to boost supply of fats. Firstly the loss of lean muscle mass as discussed above. That is why recently both ACSM and HPB has included resistance training as part of their exercise recommendation. It is to defend muscle loss and therefore prevent increase in fats. The second thing is that when we are hungry, our senses will scan for energy dense food also known as foods high in fats. Fried and creamy dishes for example will look more appealing. Our ears will recognize food being fried and our sense of smell will alert us of this types of food. All this information will be fed to the brain and overwhelms the decision making component of the brain to choose these types of unhealthy food to regain energy balance quickly. Healthy foods, on the other hand, will not be picked up by our 'sense radar'. Thirdly, to ensure that fuel storage is maximized, mobilization of fats for physical activity has been made difficult. For example, the body's preferred fuel for exercise is glucose, not fats. As mentioned, glucose supply in the body is enough to power physical activity between 90 to 120 minutes. By that time, we will be too exhausted to continue. Also, fats are only optimally mobilized at a low level intensity, specifically 60 – 70 % of our MHR. From my observation, a majority of us tend to exercise too hard or too fast so much so we tend to stop prematurely. A good physical activity is brisk walking but this has to be done at a longer duration like 2 hours. Lastly, the brain, upon sensing a caloric drop either through increased physical activity or reduction in caloric intake, will lower the metabolic rate so much so that it may cancel any benefits of short spurts of exercise. Hope that will explain why some of us experience no change in weight even though we have been cutting down a little on our food or went for a short workout. To be effective in achieving caloric deficit (where caloric expenditure is greater than intake) and therefore weight loss, the exercise has to be significant enough. As can be see, the body will go through a lot of trouble to ensure that fat storage is not harmed and quite the opposite, multiply. So in a way those who have gained weight is testament to how well the human body works.

I like to think of the difficulty to weight loss like a one way street where it is very easy to gain unhealthy weight but very difficult to lose it and as already explained above, it is just how the human body has been engineered. That being said, there are a couple of tricks that can be adopted to expedite weight loss. One way I find very effective is to do a lot of sit ups. It is not so much to develop 'durians' or 'abs' but I find that the muscles around the tummy firms up so much so that expansion due to over eating will cause discomfort. In other words, it can make us experience an artificial feeling of being full. However, when I mention a lot of sit ups, I mean a lot of sit ups and the amount differ from one to another. I would not like to put a number down but rather focus on the feeling, that is, there should be some soreness to be felt at the tummy region the next day. This is called Delayed Onset Muscle Soreness or DOMS, where the muscles actually experience micro tear in the muscle fibre in order for it to grow or become denser. Common questions to be asked about the tummy region for those who are overweight is whether we can target weight loss area to specific body parts and whether we can 'grow abs'. For the first part of the question, it is unlikely to target weight loss area to specific body parts. When our body experience weight loss, our body has priority as to where to take the fats from. The first region where fats will be taken from is the face and the last place, for men, tummy, for ladies, the bum.

Exercise for Weight Gain

Unbeknownst to many, exercising for the purpose of gaining weight is much tougher than losing it. For those whose BMI is below 18.5, exercise should mainly focus on strength training complemented with a high protein diet. Aerobic exercise should also be attempted but in shorter duration so as to minimize greater muscle loss. But the common misconception to increase weight is by eating unhealthy food. Doing so will only increase the unhealthy weight in one body, not to mention fuelling unhealthy eating habits to one's lifestyle. My students like to give suggestions on how to increase one's weight; to eat fast food every day. Clearly, I had to correct them each time for this misconception.

To increase healthy weight is to increase lean muscle mass. This can be achieved by doing resistance training either with free or assisted weights. However, for it to be effective, the repetitions in a set has to be reduced to between 5 to 8, to exhaustion. This will stimulate muscle growth. From my observations however, many girls are reluctant to do weights training. Their concern with this type of training was the aesthetic outlook where they would certainly not want to look like professional female bodybuilders they so often see on magazine covers. This is obviously an almost impossible task to perform because professional body builders take many training hours to perfect their body shape, not to mention this is complemented with a diet of supplements to achieve great gains in muscle mass. For weight gain to be observed, enough rest must also be observed where at least 7-8 hours of sleep ensures the body have sufficient time to recuperate from weight lifting.

Conclusion

Exercise can be simple or complex. Different people take exercise to different levels. The important thing is that it should be taken at a level that is comfortable and convenient to the individual. For a housewife who brisk walks 20 minutes to the market and brisk walk another 20 minutes to return home, that can be considered her daily exercise. For the person who takes a more serious approach to exercise, it could mean driving 20 minutes to East Coast Park to jog an hour along the beach. The important thing is that it must be convenient for the person to enjoy exercising. The moment we feel that exercise might be a drag, the chances of the doing it again in the future becomes minimal. Sustainability is key and the key to sustainability is incorporating it into our daily lifestyle. It is unrealistic to continue with current practices or lifestyle while trying to introduce new ones. Something has to be sacrificed. To squeeze in that one hour of brisk walk, it could mean giving up an hour of TV time. The point is, whatever it is that needs to be sacrificed, it should be an unhealthy habit or things that are worth to be forgone. Another point that is worth mentioning here is that in our busy schedule, we have to rush to exercise. Sometimes the workout can be as little as 10 minutes but little is better than nothing.

For one's commitment to exercise, also bear in mind not to get injured. All forms of precaution must be taken to ensure that injury can be avoided, for example,

- having enough fluids before, during and after the exercise bout,
- warming up and cooling down,
- using equipment and facilities that are not faulty,
- not exercising at least 3 hours after a main meal,
- having enough rest in between exercises,
- not exercising when already injured.
- when outdoors, avoid exercising when the sun is shining brightly or when it's raining and when there is risk of lightning.

Chapter 5

Stress

Living in Singapore can be highly stressful. Many of us somewhat perform a juggling act while keeping our sanity intact. Central to our lives is our job where we spend most of our waking moments. Then we have other commitments like family, friends, finances, housing etc. But have we actually paused and asked ourselves - what we are doing all this for or at what point of our lives are we at or are we happy with ourselves right now? I'm sure we all have and at different time, arrive at different conclusions.

Stress in small or manageable amount is actually necessary in our daily life and routine. Stress starts to be problematic when it becomes overwhelming and one finds himself or herself unable to cope with it. Prolonged exposure to high level of stress can manifest itself physically like high blood pressure and stomach ulcers. Psychologically, one may even experience anxiety attacks and even depression. Having good physical and social health would not ensure good overall health if the stress level is also not manageable. Therefore managing stress is important in the overall maintenance of health.

A quick web check in salaryexplorer.com reveals that Singapore is the third most stressful country to work in. This placing is said to be behind Switzerland and United Arab Emirates and among all the job categories, the occupation of teaching ranked third as the most stressful job. This job, which ranked behind those in quality control and telecommunications, is something my wife and I can sometimes relate to. Occasionally we find ourselves sitting on our bed, working on our own individual laptops way through the night as our children played outside. Indeed, a teacher's job typically involve lesson planning and teaching, marking assignments, setting papers, planning events, attending meetings and professional courses, as well as looking after the well-being and holistic development of the students under his or her charge, are part of the work of a teacher.

The World Health Organisation defines mental health as a state of well-being in which every individual realizes his or her own potential, can cope with the normal stress of life, can work productively and fruitfully, and is able to make a contribution to her or his community. Based on this definition alone, we score very well in the last component of making a contribution to the community, in this case, our work targets. But not all of us are able to work productively consistently. We can cope with the normal stress of life but how many of us have actually realized our potentials. Have we actually determined what our potentials are? I would like to think that it is just a simple matter of happiness. So how happy are we as Singaporeans? According to happyplanetindex.org, Singapore HPI or Happy Planet Index is 39.8. This index ranked us in the 90th placing out of 151 countries. This is definitely not good as this ranking shows that we are below the median or we are actually in the second half of the index.

Managing stress is therefore something that is important to ensure a better quality of life. As teachers, we see many students who manage stress well but others have poor stress management which caused them to 'lose-it' This is where they express themselves through irrational behaviour like anger and shouting. Quite understandably, students have to cope with a myriad of issues like studies, Co-Curriculum Activity or CCA and sometimes the things that help them cope with stress, like friends and family can add pressure instead.

On the topic of maintaining mental health, being positive certainly helps a lot. As the common saying goes, being positive is like looking at the cup half full instead of half empty. In other words, feeling grateful for what we have instead of what we have not, truly gives a positive perspective in life. For example, being in a safe country like Singapore amidst a backdrop of countries hit by natural disasters and going through political and social instabilities, we should feel grateful and fortunate to be living in this city-state. This feeling of gratitude can easily felt with a simple thought that we have our own families and a roof over our heads. A stable job is another reason for most of us to be grateful about life. There are many others but ultimately, it is important to feel sincere about feeling grateful. Feeling a sense of let-down after having failed to do a task can be daunting, however, when we look back and take stock of what we have achieved so far, the feeling of contentment will override the initial feeling of underachieving and often gives me a sense of consolation.

If I may share my experience at coping with stress, at times, I get caught in situations which cause me to feel emotional. I likened it to a temporary state of depression. As soon as I realize that I am going through this, my coping mechanism kicks in. For this, I have a two prong approach. One is to recall my past significant achievements in life and the other is the skill sets that I have. These are my assets and it is something that can never be taken away. They are also quite unique in a sense that these assets are what defines me and essentially, differentiate me from others. They work as confidence boosters and helps me in times of need to increase my self-esteem. I think everyone has these assets and it is important that everyone recognize how unique they truly are as these exact features make them special. So I think it is important that we do our best to achieve something in life and develop our skill sets. These can be in many areas, the most important of which is education, where we must strive to achieve the highest educational qualification that we can. In terms of skill sets, we can look into the aesthetics for example the ability to play musical instruments, act or dance. Other unique capabilities one can acheive is in sports where this will highlight the individual as a unique person from society. Although it may take time and effort to develop skills in sports, bear in mind that the more unique the skill set and the higher the level of achievement, the more impervious the individual can become towards life challenges.

That being said, each of us has our own unique way of de-stressing. There are those that are healthy and those that are not. Two very unhealthy ways of de-stressing is through emotional eating and emotional spending. It is a common behavior or practice that when we do well in something we would want to celebrate by going out for a good meal. While to me this is quite acceptable because we do not always achieve successes or promotions, turning our attention to food to make us feel good can be quite a different matter altogether. This type of association or relationship with food can increase the size of our waistline. This is because we depend on food to improve the negative state of our emotions instead of looking at food as a means of sustenance to live healthily. If we do have such a relationship with food, we must control ourselves by first changing our perception of food as just another element, like air, that we need to survive. It is imperative to understand that healthy food is a function of a healthy state of body and mind.

There are many healthy ways of de-stressing. The two common ways are socially and physically. Talking about our problems is perhaps the most common and most effective way of relieving stress. Our listeners can include family members, friends and even professionals like counsellors or psychiatrists. Some turn to religious leaders to air their problems. Choosing the right listener is important. A wrong listener is one who may give the wrong advice, or worse, expose our problems in the open, leaving us embarrassed and vulnerable. As teachers, we see it sometimes in our students. That is why we recommend they consult their parents about their problems or their teachers or school counsellors. Many also, including myself, turn to exercise to de-stress. Working the muscles and heart has been found in many studies to alleviate symptoms of stress. Why not combine social and physical for that double-whammy effect? That is, to exercise in a group. I get my fix every Saturday morning by going cycling with a few friends. I regularly jog with my wife too. During these bouts of exercise, we talk about work-related issues, family challenges and others. Sometimes we may feel too tired to exercise but most of the time after the exercise we will feel better and not regret the decision to do it. I call it the 'Maryam Phenomenon'. Maryam is my 17 year old daughter. Every weekend I take my children swimming and Maryam is the one to pull the longest face saying that she's too tired and asks to be excused. In all instances, I remained steadfast in my decision and insist she finish her laps. At the end of the session, I will find her perk up, smiling, laughing and joking around with her siblings. It may seem perplexing to see a sudden drastic change in behavior but there is a perfectly good scientific evidence to this. When we exercise, a hormone called endorphin is secreted into our bloodstream. Endorphin is "feel good" hormone, a type of natural, self-induced drug. And like all drugs, it is addictive. That explains why people continue to exercise and in some instances, they will feel depress when they don't. This phenomenon is called 'Runners' High'.

Unfortunately, all that have been discussed above do not effectively solve the problems as they just address the symptoms. To tackle stress, we must strike at the source. We need to identify what actually causes the stress and resolve it. For example, a person who is afraid of spiders will leave the room when a spider suddenly appears. Removing himself or herself from the room will relieve him of the stress at that moment but the same reaction is expected in future encounters. To effectively and permanently remove the stress, that person has to face his or her fears. Action may include studying the creature's anatomy and physiology and its place in the eco-system, kind of what spider enthusiasts will do. When the perception changes that spiders are actually beautiful creatures of nature, the problem can be permanently overcomed. Similarly, if we have issues at work or at home, identify what actually causes it instead of walking away from it. Sometimes it can be a simple case of miscommunication. Sometimes we may need a little time before facing the issue, it's alright. Sometimes we need assistance from others, like a mediator. Whatever it is, suffering in silence is the never good and can lead to clinical depression which can escalate to mental disorder. To cope with overwhelming stress others may resort to substance abuse like drugs. Drinking is another way many try to cope with stress. Smokers often use cigarette as a means to de-stress and that is the reason why quitting can be impossible because smoking is part of the coping strategies employed. The last three examples of coping with stress are highly negative and harms the body in the long run and must be discontinued as soon as possible. Going for a holiday is a great way to 'get away from things' but like what is said above, it does not solve the problem, just the symptoms. Facing our fears and problems remain the best way to get over our stress.

Another effective method of de-stressing that is more passive in nature is meditation. This is the most convenient way of managing stress as it requires almost no preparation and can be done almost anywhere with very little or no equipment, although a room where you can be alone in and a little soothing and calm music can help. Some go to the extent of burning scented wood or oil to increase the mood. Meditation is essentially some alone time where one empties the mind and subsequently fills it up with images that can calm the human spirit like the beach or a waterfall. Deep breathing and consciously loosening the muscles at the shoulders and neck can help towards achieving a calm state of mind. It is amazing what just five minutes of meditation can do to the mind. But for meditation to work well, it should be done regularly. Establishing a routine is important as our brain works well when there is a set pattern. Elite athletes often use this method to prepare themselves for competition and it has proven to help performance.

The very first step in managing stress is recognizing when it becomes overwhelming. This is quite easy to detect. For most of us, it means an increase in our heart rate and breathing can get more rapid and deeper.

Some of us experience perspiration, especially in the palm of our hands. Our muscles may also stiffen, especially at the shoulder and neck region. In severe cases, blurred vision may be experienced.

Psychologically, one may not be able to focus on anything at all when under stress. There could be a delay in reaction and verbal responses may not make much sense too. When one experiences such symptoms, it is important that we first make a conscious effort to recognize that we are in a stressful situation and the next thing to do is to calm ourselves down. This can be done by doing a simple exercise of firstly taking a deep breath, stiffening our shoulders while clenching our fists and secondly breathing out slowly while relaxing the shoulders and opening out our fists. Do this several times. What is important is not to continue to be in such an acidic environment. And I have come so far to learn that making decision when under a lot of stress almost always end up in having to turn back this decision.

Indeed, stress is a double edge sword. It has its place in our lives and is here to stay and should stay. A life that has no stress is bad for the human spirit and have detrimental effect as well. Managing stress is an important skill to have and develop upon to better manage our lives. While many of us develop coping mechanism quite naturally and incidentally, some of us do not and are caught off guard and fall prey to mental illnesses. A good mental state of health together with social and physical health is what is desired to ensure quality living.

Chapter 6

Socialize

Among all living creatures on earth, homosapiens or humans have the most advanced and sophisticated communication ability, be it verbal or non-verbal and it is still developing at a very rapid pace with the aid of technology. It is only expected then that humans must live with each other and isolating a member from the rest is not only unnatural but cruel. Over time, cultures, practices and rules have blanketed civilizations and societies to ensure harmonious living environments. And in oder to live harmoniously, awareness in individual or group differences is an important skill to have, not only for safety but also overall health. This skill, if accompanied with the ability to relate and work well with others cans significantly ensure success for the individual. Thus is the importance and standing of social well-being in the health equation.

Wikianswers define social well-being as involving a person's relationships with others and how that person communicates, interacts and socializes with other people. It can also relate to how people make friends and whether they have a sense of belonging. For example, going to the movies with friends is being social. Singapore's Ministry of Education's Social and Emotional Learning framework outlines five components, one of which is Relationship Management which directly places an emphasis on how important working and learning with others is. Teachers equip students, our future, on how to communicate, work cooperatively, negotiate, refuse and manage conflicts, seek and provide help as well as engage and build relationships. Educational packages to teach these skills will hopefully help students become healthier and more importantly functional and well-adjusted adults. From another angle, Howard Gardner, the proponent of The Theory of Multiple Intelligence, included interpersonal skill as part of the nine intelligences a person should have. He asserts, as reported in Wikipedia, that people with high interpersonal intelligence are characterized by their sensitivity to others' moods, feelings, temperaments and motivations and their willingness to cooperate as part of a group. Those with this intelligence communicate effectively and empathize easily with others and may either be leaders or followers. They typically learn best working with others and often enjoy discussions and debates.

In practical terms, social well-being to me is about having a strong personal support system with family and friends. In the event of hardship, be it at work or of a personal nature, such support system will be able to help overcome challenges and continue living fulfilling lives. This is because events in our lives can turn out sour at times when we are least prepared. Depending on with whom the relationships are established with and the nature of the tragedy, some will turn to family, others to friends, many others to colleagues while the rest, to professionals. Whatever it is, problems are most often best managed by seeking opinions and advice from others whom we trust. Moreover, most often than not, family is said to be party with the least likelihood of betraying trust. That is why family relationships must be first and foremost be protected and developed to a level that personal differences and external challenges cannot disrupt the cordial relationship among members. For that reason, many governments have declared that family is the building blocks of society, including Singapore. Here are some tips adapted from Dr. Laura Markham (online) on how to build strong, happy and close family.

- Having a meal together. Dinner would be a good time for weekdays and try to include lunch and even breakfast over the weekend. This type of get together allows members to discuss issues with their guards down. Most often, meal time is relaxed and therefore a good time to ask favors from one another. Communication is at its best at these sessions.

- Parents have to be emotionally present for their children or even each other at the end of a hard day's work. This is an especially difficult task when parents themselves are tired after work but doing so can make or break a child.

- Children may seem that they don't like rules but research suggest otherwise. They actually thrive on routines and structure. A predictable routine allows children to feel safe, develop self-discipline and gain a sense of mastery in handling their lives. This is so true. I love to ask my students when school re-opens after a long holiday whether they enjoyed their holidays. Most would replied that it was boring as they didn't have much to do and sheepishly admit that they are happier in school.

- Play together, be it indoors or outdoors. Parents should try things that their children enjoy playing like electronic games, board games, party games, card games, sports etc. and introduce them to games that they want their children to learn like traditional games. Playing silly like giving horse rides to their young ones is a great way to create bonding not only to the toddler but the siblings who are watching.

Other tips Dr Markham gave include having regular family meetings, helping siblings overcome rivalries, making the home a safe heaven or sanctuary and discovering the great outdoors together.

Other than the given tips, I have found a couple of effective practices one can adopt in their lives. This refer to performing prayers together and teaching our own children. The ritualistic and solemn act of praying somehow instil in all the family members a type of group discipline. Children naturally accepts their parents' leadership in this area where they need guidance in, most of whom cannot claim that they are experts in, unlike the electronic world where they reign as knowledge and skill masters of the house. Even though they may seem uninterested in religion, they do have that moral compass in them to tell themselves that what they are doing is good and necessary and who better to equip them than their own parents. Teaching our own children entails passing down our own skills and knowledge of our own interest and passion or getting an expert to teach them the things that we enjoyed doing when we were young or we were good in. This should be done in a structured way and to see the results it should be conducted regularly and consistently. I find doing this particularly helpful in building bonds as it increases communication between parents and children when the former give guidance and feedback. I often advise parents who want to enroll their children in enrichment programmes to choose the ones that they were engaged in when they were young or they are still enjoying. I find it rather rewarding seeing the 'fruits of my labour' after many years of coaching my children simple things like playing chess, swimming and playing musical instruments. I don't consider myself an expert, I just teach them the basic skills, enough for them to be independent in these areas. My wife also gets them involved in traditional dance form, an activity she used to do when she was young. All these I feel has helped our family closer and more dynamic.

Friends are also important to ensure good social health. I think we should have close friends that we should keep till old age. They may be our school friends, colleagues or ex-colleagues, friends we meet at seminars and meetings etc. Sometimes we meet them at regular intervals like weekend games or once in a while for a meal. Such gatherings can be refreshing as we discuss matters that are usually of the same interests which may be far away from the mundane tasks we usually toil at work. A reunion is a great way to reconnect with old friends and relive the glorious past and one should make all the effort to attend such gatherings. My wife and I sometimes take time out from our duties as parents to have dinner with friends. It's a great way to re-charge after a hectic week at work. Not only that, sometimes she would ask me if she could go out with her girlfriends, either from work, ex-colleagues, ex-schoolmates, cousins or even ex-students. I always encourage her to do so. While my wife's outings with friends are ad-hoc. I meet up with my cycling buddies weekly over the weekend. Working out together and having coffee after that us rejuvenating, something all members of the group look forward to at the end of the work week. Every year, our family would go for a short holiday with another two families who have about as many children as us. We have been doing this for many years and we call ourselves Travelling With Kids or TWK for short. We have grown quite close over the years and often confide in each other, parents and children, over almost everything under the sun. We find such relationship very uplifting to our personal growth. Web friends such as those from Facebook, Twitter, and Instagram are good too but often lack the dimension and depth as physical ones. In times of need, other than family and the workplace, friends can be a strong pillar of support. They can help us overcome grief and even introduce us to new network of friends to help us move on quickly. However, friends can also be a source of trouble and stress, thus it is important to choose friends wisely and sometimes, if differences are not able to be resolved, relationship may be more detrimental if continued.

Social skills are important to have and it is worth spending time and effort to learn and develop or even re-learn new ones. This is because, in most, if not all, instances, working together towards a common goal is far more effective doing it in a group than alone. The adage, 'Too many cooks spoil the soup' should be entirely replaced with 'Many heads are better than one'. But this is not only about working but also play. Players in team games can tell us that for a team to be effective and successful, it is about accepting each other's weaknesses, capitalizing on individual strengths and every member working hard to improve and contribute. So, if all of us belong to teams or groups of friends and have strong, grounded relationships with family members, life will not only be healthy but also fulfilling beyond imagination.

Chapter 7

Uniformed Progression

Human being's ability to adapt is simply amazing. In the area of Sports Science, athletes training in high altitude simply takes about 2 weeks to acclimatize to new environment at which point their bodies produce more red blood cells to boost hemoglobin concentrations in the body to make up for the lack of oxygen in the air. This will allow the body to absorb more oxygen needed by the working muscles. So when they return to sea levels for competition, they will have an advantage when the body with greater count of red blood cells is able to absorb the abundant amount of oxygen in the air as compared to that in high altitude. But the effects also lasts about two weeks as the body re-adjust to the current level of oxygen concentration in the air. The lesson to learn from this example is that our bodies respond to changes in the environment and the changes are slow and not permanent. To change, we would have to undergo a different experience which the body and mind may not like. Therefore, expect resistance when introducing new actions to improve health through, as mentioned in the previous chapters, a healthy diet, having enough rest, exercising, socializing and managing stress. This is due to the human body's pre-disposition to accumulate fats and remain at homeostasis or remaining in the comfort zone for as long as possible.

In my experience, two issues needs to be addressed first, our value system and motivation level. Briefly, we need to prioritize health first and see it as the key towards happiness and all other priorities such as career and money. The next action is to find the right motivation to do the right things and as discussed before, internal motivation is superior to external ones. Whatever it is, when introducing changes, especially healthy ones, it is best to include all, for example, just exercising alone will not be effective to lose weight.

In this chapter, we will learn the mechanism involved in making successful changes and forming new habits as well as discover why most of the time making resolution, almost always fail. First, we will need to understand that our brain has a conscious and a subconscious domain. Our conscious brain is responsible for making decisions while we are awake and alert while our subconscious brain is basically our reflex action, where decisions are mostly automatic and goes by feeling. To see how powerful each of these domains are, take a look at the data below;

	CONSCIOUS	SUBCONSCIOUS
Percentage of brain used	17	83
Control of daily action & thinking	2% – 4%	96% - 98%
Processing speed	7km/hr	60 000km/hr
Processing volume	2000 bits/sec	400 billion bits/sec

Subconscious thinking basically rule our daily life and dictate our actions. The part of the brain where subconscious thinking reside is called the amygdala. Understanding the amygdala is key towards making successful changes so read on.

The amygdala works like an air-con thermostat. When room temperature is above the one set, it will start blowing cold air. When room is cool enough, cold air stops blowing. Similarly, when the amygdala senses change, it reacts by sending signal to other parts of the brain which causes stress, anxiety, doubt and fear. This feeling is the one that prevents a caveman from entering a dark cave or eating an unrecognizable fruit. The same subconscious mechanism that is used to protect human can now hold us back from achieving our goals and targets by telling us to stay inside our comfort zones like eating the same types food and sticking to the same leisure activity instead of trying on new ones. For example, John loves beef *rendang* (a typical Malay Singaporean dish which is spicy) and when the Malay stall at his workplace serves this dish every Wednesday, he would order it. However one day, he decided to stop having it because he knows that it is not healthy. So he starts to look at other dishes available but whatever dish that he shortlisted, especially the healthier ones, the amygdala sends a feeling of fear that it would not satisfy his hunger or he would not enjoy lunch that day. Chances are he would revert back to his old favourite dish, beef *rendang*.

Many of us have been in a similar situation as the example above and the good news is that it does not apply only to negative examples. Those who have been practising healthy habits will report discomfort when having to take on unhealthier ones or being unable to continue with healthy regiments. A friend of mine even tells me that he will fall ill if he stops exercising. This is because practices have been ingrained into the subconscious such that it has become second nature. Such habits can be cultivated but will take time, effort, through several processes which will be discussed in the following paragraphs.

A technique that should be used together with the action plan is called mental re-training which involves visualization in the head. Many researches have been done in this area and scientists have concluded that it actually improves performance by preparing our muscles to the specific action that is to be completed. When a PET Scan was conducted on visualization exercise, Scientist found that the brain respond similarly to actual and imagined events. As we imagine, the brain creates pathways to support and process new goals. The brain will eventually accept the fact and makes things easier. Visualization can be done by stating each desire and acting it out in the mind with passion and emotion. It should be done in moments where and when concentration is the highest. It need not be in a quiet atmosphere like in a dark quiet room, it can simply be on the way to work, in the MRT or after a meal etc. Visualizing exercise takes a very short time of between 30 – 60 seconds but it should be done 4 – 5 times a day and for it to be effective this exercise should be repeated for a period of 26 – 30 days.

Regarding what to visualize, images of success and enjoyment in the process of achieving that success would be suitable. For example

- imagining a slim or muscular figure
- eating healthy food and enjoying it
- exercising and having fun
- being in bed by 10pm to get the restful 7-8 hours rest etc

So it actually helps one's mind to cultivate a healthy living when posters of athletic pleasing people or models are put up as posters as this greatly enforces the visualization process. They also function as reminders of the many visualization exercises to be conducted each day. A month of mental re-training can re-set the internal thermostat or the amygdala. It allows goals to be achieved with less resistance. However it takes about 100 days or 3 months for a new habit to be cultivated. Consistency and persistency is important. Flexibility should also be incorporated for example, it is alright to regress once in a while for example having an ice-cream treat after many days or a week of healthy eating, just as long as there is general progression throughout the period.

Researchers have stated that it takes a hundred days to form a new habit and that it is possible to cultivate and adopt a mental toughness within ourselves. The technique used by sports coaches or trainers is called mental re-training. The process involves re-training the subconscious mind to new images in the head to replace the old ones that are holding us back. It starts with goal setting.

Exercise Planning Using the SMART Method

Educators always say to their students, "If you fail to plan, you plan to fail." The SMART method, S – specific, M – measurable, A – achievable, R – Realistic, T – Time-bound, is a very effective way to ensure results. If our aim is to improve our fitness, it is not enough just to go out there and workout. The guide below will show how. To improve fitness, firstly we need to know our starting fitness level. This can be done in many ways for example taking a 2km walk test where at the end of the test, participants will find out the level of fitness achieved like, Bronze, Silver or Gold. To improve health, our health indicators like weight, BMI, blood pressure, body fat percentage, body age, etc needs to be determined first. A good fitness or health plan should be accompanied by record keeping. This will help us understand the amount of improvement that we have made or whether the exercise programme is effective, and if not, introduce further measures. Try to write down the exercise plan as much as possible. This will keep us focused to achieving our goals. Studies shows that visual tracking is more effective than those that are just kept in our minds.

Specific

For fitness, to be specific could be to improve running fitness or muscular strength. For health it could be to improve blood pressure or body fat percentage. For diet it could focus on having more regular meals. For rest it could mean having enough sleep.

Measurable

It is important that the fitness or health component chosen to improve on is measurable. For example, running fitness can be measured by distance, time or even award. The target could be to run 2.4km from 18 minutes to 15 minutes, increase running distance at the stadium from 8 laps in 30 minutes to 10 laps in the same amount of time or getting the silver award in the 2km walk test from the bronze award in the Sports for Life fitness assessment. For health, it could be lowering the blood pressure from 140/90 to 120/80 or reduce body fat percentage from 20% to 18%.

Achievable & Realistic

These two components have just about the same objectives. As the word suggest, we need to evaluate if the targets we set ourselves is something that can be achieved. In other words, a reality check is in order. For example, it is not realistic to set a target of running a full marathon when we've not even attempted several 21km run. Of course this person can complete the whole marathon but in what way? If more than half of the distance is completed by walking and having to take medical leave the next day to recover, then truly the target is not a realistic one.

Time Bound

Yet another important component to the planning equation, having time factored into our goals, will make planning very effective. It is good to have three time frames, short, medium and long. For example, a runner would want to improve his 2.4km run test timing from 18 to 15 minutes in one year period for the short term goal. For the medium frame, he may want to take part in two to three 10km run and at least one 21km run. And for the long term goal is to run his first marathon in five years' time. For health improvement, it could mean lowering the blood pressure or body fat within a year.

On the whole, when all the components have been factored in, it would look something like this; To reduce body fat percentage by 2% in one year or to be able to shave 3 minutes in the 2.4km fitness test run in 12 months time. Or to have seven hours of sleep five days of the week in six months time. For diet it could be eating brown rice once a week by three months time. After the goals have been established, the next step is to focus on the action plan. For exercise, we can use the FITT and the training principles mentioned in the earlier chapters.

Do take note that a health plan must be as personal as possible, that is, it should not be adopted from others as everybody's lifestyle is different from one another, even twins! Write this down and display it prominently. It will help us focus on our targets. This approach can be applied to many other fields including studies, sports, etc.

Switching to a healthier lifestyle is essentially about changing habits, which is an arduous task. Those who have asked me what they should do to be healthier wants to know what they should eat or how to exercise. But now we know that it's actually about forming new healthier habits and the key towards changing habits is actually re-shaping our value systems. This is actually the last of the four pillars of effective change to a healthier lifestyle. The first three being motivation, knowledge of health and action.

The first step to re-shaping our value system is identifying all our priorities. Write down ten priorities we have in life and then rank them from 1 to 10 in order of importance. These could be family, career, religion, money, health etc. If health is on the top three priorities, then it is good. If not, then we have to move it up there by rationalization. This can be done by convincing ourselves that health impacts the other priorities. For example, many of us may put career or family as one of the top three but if our health is poor we will not be able to perform our roles well in these two domains. If our immunity is low due to a sedentary lifestyle and poor diet, we will fall ill often and as a result may be an absent family member frequently. As a parent, we would not want to burden the family with health cost or not being around much due to medical consultations and treatments. In fact, a fit and healthy person automatically is a better mother, father, son, daughter, worker, soldier, worshipper and let us know forget the famous adage, 'Health is Wealth'.

This book has equipped us with the four pillars of adopting a healthier lifestyle; Value System, Motivation, Knowledge & Action, in order of importance. Together with the DRESS UP approach, it will help us form lasting habits to lead healthier lifestyles which in turn will improve the quality of life, which is all that we really actually want but as discussed, not easy to achieve. Just remember that what we do today will pay off tomorrow, the harder the effort, the greater the reward. We have to fight the survival mode of hoarding fats by being active, eating healthily and having enough rest. This battle must rage on till our golden years. Those who are losing the fight, get up, resist and overcome and those who are in control, continue and be an inspiration to others, for at the rate we are going, we are losing the fight badly. May I wish all my readers all the success in the journey to a better quality of life for all to reap.